It's easy to get lost in the cancer world

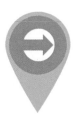

Let NCCN Guidelines for Patients® be your guide

✓ Step-by-step guides to the cancer care options likely to have the best results

✓ Based on treatment guidelines used by health care providers worldwide

✓ Designed to help you discuss cancer treatment with your doctors

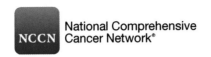

National Comprehensive
Cancer Network®

NCCN Guidelines for Patients® are developed by the National Comprehensive Cancer Network® (NCCN®)

NCCN

✓ An alliance of leading cancer centers across the United States devoted to patient care, research, and education

Cancer centers that are part of NCCN:
NCCN.org/cancercenters

NCCN Clinical Practice Guidelines in Oncology (NCCN Guidelines®)

✓ Developed by experts from NCCN cancer centers using the latest research and years of experience

✓ For providers of cancer care all over the world

✓ Expert recommendations for cancer screening, diagnosis, and treatment

Free online at
NCCN.org/guidelines

NCCN Guidelines for Patients

✓ Present information from the NCCN Guidelines in an easy-to-learn format

✓ For people with cancer and those who support them

✓ Explain the cancer care options likely to have the best results

Free online at
NCCN.org/patientguidelines

These NCCN Guidelines for Patients are based on the NCCN Guidelines® for Breast Cancer, Version 2.2022 – December 20, 2021.

NCCN Foundation seeks to support the millions of patients and their families affected by a cancer diagnosis by funding and distributing NCCN Guidelines for Patients. NCCN Foundation is also committed to advancing cancer treatment by funding the nation's promising doctors at the center of innovation in cancer research. For more details and the full library of patient and caregiver resources, visit NCCN.org/patients.

National Comprehensive Cancer Network (NCCN) / NCCN Foundation
3025 Chemical Road, Suite 100
Plymouth Meeting, PA 19462
215.690.0300

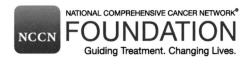

NATIONAL COMPREHENSIVE CANCER NETWORK®
FOUNDATION
Guiding Treatment. Changing Lives.

NCCN Guidelines for Patients are supported by funding from the NCCN Foundation®

To make a gift or learn more, please visit NCCNFoundation.org/donate
or e-mail PatientGuidelines@NCCN.org.

Brem Foundation

The Brem Foundation teaches women about the need for personalized screening, opens access to breast care for women in need, and advocates for public policies that increase women's opportunities to screen for breast cancer. The Brem Foundation prides itself on reaching women from all socio-economic backgrounds and has made social determinants of health a large focus in all of its work. bremfoundation.org

With additional support from Dr. Wui-Jin Koh

In honor of Judy Anne Hanada Koh

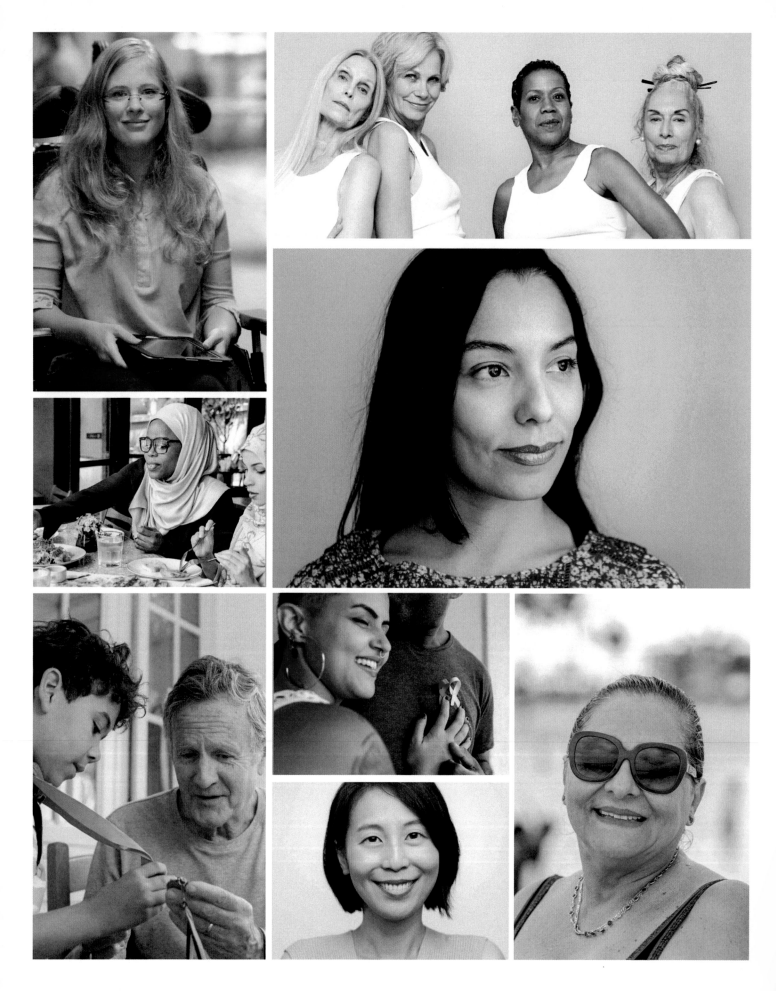

Contents

6   Breast cancer basics

10   Testing for breast cancer

25   Breast cancer staging

31   Treatment overview

52   The breast after surgery

57   Stages 1, 2, and 3A

67   Stage 3

76   Recurrence

80   Inflammatory breast cancer

88   Making treatment decisions

101 Words to know

106 NCCN Contributors

107 NCCN Cancer Centers

109 Index

1
Breast cancer basics

7   **The breast**

8   **Breast cancer**

8   **How breast cancer spreads**

9   **Key points**

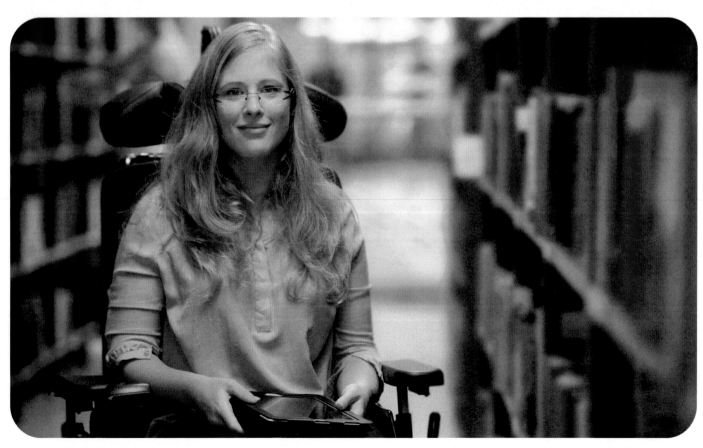

Anyone can develop breast cancer. Invasive breast cancer is cancer that has spread from the milk ducts or milk glands into the breast tissue or nearby lymph nodes.

The breast

The breast is an organ and a gland found on the chest. The breast is made of milk ducts, fat, nerves, lymph and blood vessels, ligaments, and other connective tissue. Behind the breast is the pectoral (chest) muscle and ribs. Muscle and ligaments help hold the breast in place.

Breast tissue contains glands that can make milk. These milk glands are called lobules. Lobules look like tiny clusters of grapes. Small tubes called ducts connect the lobules to the nipple to deliver breast milk.

The ring of darker breast skin is called the areola. The raised tip within the areola is called the nipple. The nipple-areola complex (NAC) is a term that refers to both parts.

Lymph is a clear fluid that gives cells water and food. It also helps to fight germs. Lymph drains from breast tissue into lymph vessels and travels to lymph nodes near your armpit (axilla). Nodes near the armpit are called axillary lymph nodes (ALNs).

The breast

The breast is a glandular organ made up of milk ducts, fat, nerves, blood and lymph vessels, and other connective tissue.

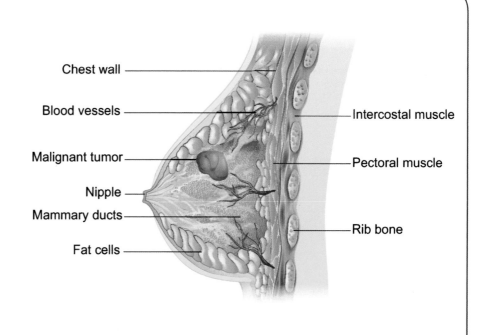

Chest wall
Blood vessels
Malignant tumor
Nipple
Mammary ducts
Fat cells
Intercostal muscle
Pectoral muscle
Rib bone

Breast cancer

Breast cancer starts in the cells of the breast. Almost all breast cancers are carcinomas. Carcinomas are cancers that start in the cells that line the inner or outer surfaces of the body.

There are different types of breast carcinoma. The most common types are either ductal or lobular.

> **Ductal carcinoma** starts in the cells that line the milk ducts. Milk ducts are thin tubes that carry milk from the lobules of the breast to the nipple. It is the most common type of breast cancer.

> **Lobular carcinoma** starts in the lobules (milk glands) of the breast.

Anyone can develop breast cancer, including males. Although there are some differences between males and females, treatment is very similar for all genders.

How breast cancer spreads

Cancer cells don't behave like normal cells. Cancer cells differ from normal cells in the following ways.

Primary tumor
Over time, cancer cells form a mass called a primary tumor.

Invasive
Cancer cells can grow into surrounding tissues. Invasive breast cancer is breast cancer that has spread from the milk ducts or milk glands (lobules) into the breast tissue or nearby lymph nodes.

Metastasis
Unlike normal cells, cancer cells can spread and form tumors in other parts of the body. Cancer that has spread to other organs is called a metastasis. In this process, cancer cells break away from the first (primary) tumor and travel through blood or lymph vessels to distant sites. Once in other sites, cancer cells may form secondary tumors.

> Cancer that has spread to a nearby body part, such as the axillary lymph nodes, is called a local metastasis. It might be referred to as local/regional disease or locally advanced disease.

> Cancer that has spread to a body part far from the primary tumor is called a distant metastasis.

Breast cancer can metastasize almost anywhere, but most commonly spread to the bones, lungs, liver, spine, or brain. Breast cancer that has metastasized to other parts of the body is still called breast cancer.

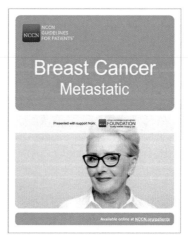

For more information on metastatic breast cancer, read the *NCCN Guidelines for Patients: Breast Cancer – Metastatic,* available at NCCN.org/ patientguidelines.

Key points

> Anyone can develop breast cancer.

> Inside breasts are lobules, ducts, fat, blood and lymph vessels, ligaments, and connective tissue. Lobules are structures that make breast milk. Ducts carry breast milk from the lobules to the nipple.

> Breast cancer often starts in the ducts or lobules and then spreads into the surrounding tissue.

> Invasive breast cancer is cancer that has grown outside the ducts or lobules into surrounding tissue. Once outside the ducts or lobules, breast cancer can spread through lymph or blood to lymph nodes or other parts of the body.

> Metastatic breast cancer has spread to distant sites in the body.

Get to know your care team and help them get to know you.

2
Testing for breast cancer

11 Test results

11 General health tests

13 Fertility

13 Preventing pregnancy

14 Blood tests

14 Imaging tests

17 Biopsy

19 Hormone receptor status

20 HER2 status

20 Biomarker testing

22 Genetic risk testing

23 Distress screening

23 Performance status

24 Key points

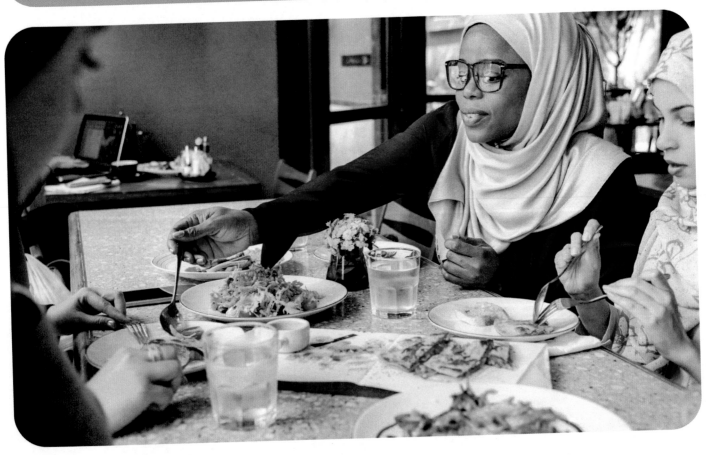

Not all invasive breast cancers are the same. Treatment planning starts with testing. Your doctor will want to gather information about the cancer you have. This chapter presents an overview of the tests you might receive and what to expect.

Test results

Results from imaging studies and biopsies will be used to determine your treatment plan. It is important you understand what these tests mean. Ask questions and keep copies of your test results. Online patient portals are a great way to access your test results.

Keep these things in mind:

> ➤ Choose a friend, family member, or peer who can drive you to appointments, provide meals, or offer emotional support during diagnosis and treatment.

> ➤ Bring someone with you to doctor visits, if possible.

> ➤ Write down questions and take notes during appointments. Don't be afraid to ask your care team questions. Get to know your care team and help them get to know you.

> ➤ Get copies of blood tests, imaging results, and reports about the specific type of cancer you have.

> ➤ Organize your papers. Create files for insurance forms, medical records, and test results. You can do the same on your computer.

> ➤ Keep a list of contact information for everyone on your care team. Add it to your phone. Hang the list on your refrigerator or keep it in a place where someone can access it in an emergency. Keep your primary care physician informed of changes to this list.

> ➤ Include in your contact list information on the exact type of cancer and stage, as well as any surgery or treatment and the date it started.

General health tests

Medical history
A medical history is a record of all health issues and treatments you have had in your life. Be prepared to list any illness or injury and when it happened. Bring a list of old and new medicines and any over-the-counter medicines, herbals, or supplements you take. Some supplements interact and affect prescriptions that your doctor may give you. Tell your doctor about any symptoms you have. A medical history, sometimes called a health history, will help determine which treatment is best for you.

Family history
Some cancers and other diseases can run in families. Your doctor will ask about the health history of family members who are blood relatives. This information is called a family history. Ask family members on both sides of your family about their health issues like heart disease, cancer, and diabetes, and at what age they were diagnosed. It important to know the specific type of cancer, or where the cancer started, and if it is in multiple locations.

Physical exam

During a physical exam, your health care provider may:

- Check your temperature, blood pressure, pulse, and breathing rate

- Check your height and weight

- Listen to your lungs and heart

- Look in your eyes, ears, nose, and throat

- Feel and apply pressure to parts of your body to see if organs are of normal size, are soft or hard, or cause pain when touched. Tell your doctor if you feel pain.

- Examine your breasts to look for lumps, nipple discharge or bleeding, or skin changes. Tell your doctor if you have noticed changes in your breast(s).

- Feel for enlarged lymph nodes in your neck and underarm. Tell your doctor if you have felt any lumps or have any pain.

For possible tests, see Guide 1.

Guide 1
Possible tests

Medical history and physical exam

Bilateral diagnostic mammogram

Breast ultrasound, as needed

Breast MRI, as needed

Biopsy with pathology review

Determine tumor status including:
- Estrogen receptor (ER) and progesterone receptor (PR) hormone receptor (HR) status
- HER2 status

Genetic counseling and/or testing if at risk for hereditary breast cancer or has triple-negative breast cancer (TNBC) (at any age)

Address fertility, birth control, and sexual health concerns

Pregnancy test in those of childbearing potential

Assess for distress

Additional imaging studies only if signs and symptoms of metastatic disease

---

Fertility

Treatment such as chemotherapy or endocrine therapy can affect your fertility, the ability to have children. If you think you want children in the future, ask your doctor how cancer and cancer treatment might change your fertility. In order to preserve your fertility, you may need to take action before starting cancer treatment. Those who want to have children in the future should be referred to a fertility specialist to discuss the options before starting treatment.

Fertility preservation is all about keeping your options open, whether you know you want to have children later in life or aren't really sure at the moment. Fertility and reproductive specialists can help you sort through what may be best for your situation.

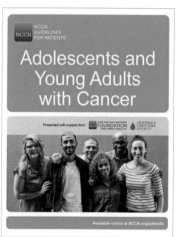

More information on fertility preservation can be found in the *NCCN Guidelines for Patients: Adolescents and Young Adults with Cancer,* available at NCCN.org/ patientguidelines.

Impaired fertility

Treatment for breast cancer might cause your fertility to be temporarily impaired or interrupted. This temporary loss of fertility is related to your age at time of diagnosis, treatment type(s), treatment dose, and treatment length. Talk to your doctor about your concerns and if you are planning a pregnancy.

Preventing pregnancy

Preventing pregnancy during treatment is important. Cancer and cancer treatment can affect the ovaries and damage sperm. Hormonal birth control may not be recommended, so ask your doctor about options such as intrauterine devices (IUDs) and barrier methods. Types of barrier methods include condoms, diaphragms, cervical caps, and the contraceptive sponge.

Those with ovaries

Those who can become pregnant will have a pregnancy test before starting treatment. Cancer treatment can hurt the baby if you are or become pregnant during treatment. Therefore, birth control to prevent pregnancy during and after treatment is recommended. If you are pregnant or breastfeeding at the time of your cancer diagnosis, certain treatments will need to be avoided.

Menstruation, menses, menstrual flow, or your "period" may stop during treatment, but often returns within 2 years after treatment in those 40 years of age and under. It is still possible to become pregnant even though you might not have a period. Therefore, birth control is recommended during and after treatment. Consult your doctor for the best time to plan a pregnancy.

Those with testicles

Cancer and cancer treatment can damage sperm. Therefore, use contraception (birth control) such as condoms to prevent pregnancy during and after cancer treatment.

Blood tests

Blood tests check for signs of disease and how well organs are working. They require a sample of your blood, which is removed through a needle placed into your vein. Some blood tests you might have are described next.

Pregnancy test

Those who can become pregnant will be given a pregnancy test before treatment begins.

Complete blood count

A complete blood count (CBC) measures the levels of red blood cells, white blood cells, and platelets in your blood. Your doctor will want to know if you have enough red blood cells to carry oxygen throughout your body, white blood cells to fight infection, and platelets to control bleeding.

Comprehensive metabolic panel

A comprehensive metabolic panel (CMP) is a test that measures 14 different substances in your blood. A CMP provides important information about how well your liver is working, and measures your electrolytes among other things. Creatinine is often part of a CMP. This test measures the health of your kidneys.

Liver function tests

Liver function tests (LFTs) look at the health of your liver by measuring chemicals that are made or processed by the liver. Levels that are too high or low signal that the liver is not working well or that cancer has spread to the liver.

Alkaline phosphatase

Alkaline phosphatase (ALP) is an enzyme found in the blood. High levels of ALP can be a sign cancer has spread to the bone or liver. A bone scan might be performed if you have high levels of ALP.

Imaging tests

Imaging tests take pictures of the inside of your body. Imaging tests show the primary tumor, or where the cancer started, and look for cancer in other parts of the body. A radiologist, who is an expert in interpreting imaging tests, will write a report and send this report to your doctor. Your doctor will discuss the results with you.

The following imaging tests are listed in alphabetical order and not in order of importance. You will not have all of these tests.

Bilateral diagnostic mammogram

A mammogram is a picture of the inside of your breast. The picture is made using x-rays. A computer combines the x-rays to make detailed pictures. Mammogram results are used to plan treatment.

Diagnostic mammograms look at specific areas of your breast, which may not be clearly seen on screening mammograms. It is used to see if there is more than one tumor and the size of the tumor(s).

Tomosynthesis or 3D mammograms are a special type of mammogram used for people with denser breast tissue to better visualize abnormalities. Other tests may include a breast MRI or ultrasound.

Bone scan

Breast cancer can spread to bones. A bone scan is an imaging test that can show if cancer has spread to your bones. This test may be used if you have bone pain, are at high risk for bone metastases, or if there are changes in certain test results. Bone scans might be used to monitor treatment. Your entire skeleton will be checked.

A bone scan uses a radiotracer. A radiotracer is a substance that releases small amounts of radiation. Before the pictures are taken, the tracer will be injected into your vein. It can take a few hours for the tracer to enter your bones. However, the test is quick and painless.

A special camera will take pictures of the tracer in your bones as it moves over your body. Areas of bone damage use more radiotracer than healthy bone and show up as bright spots on the pictures. Bone damage can be caused by cancer, cancer treatment, previous injuries, or other health problems. These tests can help identify areas that might need further testing.

Bone x-ray

An x-ray uses low-dose radiation to take one picture at a time. A tumor changes the way radiation is absorbed and will show up on the x-ray. X-rays are also good at showing bone problems. Your doctor may order x-rays if your bones hurt or were abnormal on a bone scan.

> Imaging and other tests are not always accurate. A multidisciplinary team should review the results.

CT scan

A computed tomography (CT or CAT) scan uses x-rays and computer technology to take pictures of the inside of the body. It takes many x-rays of the same body part from different angles. All the images are combined to make one detailed picture.

A CT scan of your chest, abdomen, and/or pelvis may be one of the tests to look for cancer. In most cases, intravenous (IV) contrast will be used.

Contrast

Contrast material is used to improve the pictures of the inside of the body. Contrast materials are not dyes, but substances that help enhance and improve the images of several organs and structures in the body. It is used to make the pictures clearer. The contrast is not permanent and will leave the body in your urine immediately after the test. The types of contrast vary but are different for CT than MRI.

Tell your doctors if you have had allergic reactions to contrast in the past, especially to iodine or to shellfish such as shrimp. This is important. You might be given medicines, such as Benadryl and prednisone, to avoid the effects of those allergies. Contrast might not be used if you have a serious allergy or if your kidneys aren't working well.

MRI

A magnetic resonance imaging (MRI) scan uses radio waves and powerful magnets to take pictures of the inside of the body. It does not use x-rays. Tell your doctor if you have any metal in your body. During the test, you will likely be asked to hold your breath for 10 to 20 seconds as the technician collects the images. Tell your doctor if you tend to have claustrophobia.

Breast MRI

If needed, a breast MRI would be used in addition to a mammogram. Contrast should be used. You will be positioned face down in the machine with your arms above your head.

Spine and brain MRI

An MRI can be used to detect breast cancer that has spread (metastasize) to your spine or brain. For a brain MRI, a device is placed around your head. For a spine MRI, no device is worn. Contrast should be used in an MRI.

PET/CT scan

A positron emission tomography (PET) scan uses a radioactive drug called a tracer. A tracer is a substance injected into a vein to see where cancer cells are in the body and if they are using sugar produced by your body to grow. Cancer cells show up as bright spots on PET scans. However, not all tumors will appear on a PET scan. Also, not all bright spots are cancer. It is normal for the brain, heart, kidneys, and bladder to be bright on PET. Inflammation or infection can also show up as a bright spot. When a PET scan is combined with CT, it is called a PET/CT scan. It may be done with one or two machines depending on the cancer center.

Sodium fluoride PET/CT

A sodium fluoride PET/CT might be used instead of a bone scan. In this test, the radiotracer is made of sodium fluoride.

FDG PET/CT

An FDG PET/CT uses a radiotracer called F-18 fluorodeoxyglucose (FDG). It is made of fluoride and a simple form of sugar called glucose. You cannot eat or drink for at least 4 hours before the scan. This scan is most helpful when other imaging results are unclear. It may help find cancer in lymph nodes and distant sites. If it clearly shows cancer in the bone, a bone scan and sodium fluoride PET/CT may not be needed. FDG PET/CT can be done at the same time as a CT used for diagnosis.

Ultrasound

An ultrasound (US) uses high-energy sound waves to form pictures of the inside of the body. This is similar to the sonogram used for pregnancy. A wand-like probe will be held and moved on your bare breast using gel. It may also be placed below your armpit. Ultrasound is painless and does not use x-rays, so it can be repeated as needed. Ultrasound is good at showing small areas of cancer that are near the skin. Sometimes, a breast ultrasound or MRI is used to guide a biopsy.

Biopsy

A biopsy is a procedure that removes a sample of tissue or fluid from the body. The sample is sent to a lab for testing. A pathologist will examine the biopsy for cancer and write a report called a pathology report. Ask questions about your biopsy results and what it means for your treatment.

Once an abnormal area has been found, your team may need to check whether a cancer is in the abnormal area. There are different types of biopsies. Some biopsies are guided using imaging, such as mammmogram, ultrasound, or MRI. The primary or main tumor is biopsied first. Other tumors or tumors in different areas may also be biopsied. You may have tissue removed from the breast, lymph nodes, or both.

Types of possible biopsies include:

> **Fine-needle aspiration (FNA) or core biopsy (CB)** uses needles of different sizes to remove a sample of tissue or fluid.

> **Incisional biopsy** removes a small amount of tissue through a cut in the skin or body.

> **Excisional biopsy** removes the entire abnormal area. This is not the preferred type of biopsy but may be necessary if other methods are not possible or when the biopsy results don't match the expected findings.

Before biopsies are performed, usually the area is injected with numbing medicine. A core needle biopsy removes more than one tissue sample. The samples are small. A "vacuum"

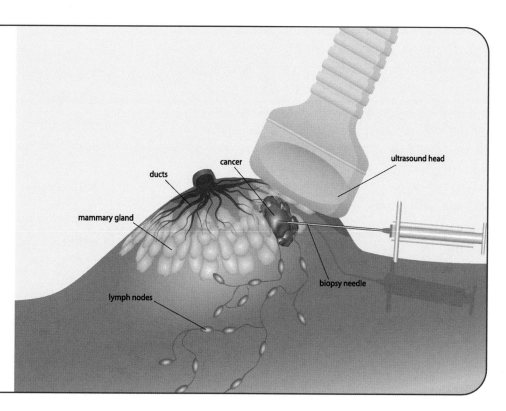

Biopsy

In a biopsy, a sample of tumor is removed. There are different types of biopsy. This image shows an ultrasound-guided needle biopsy.

ducts

cancer

mammary gland

ultrasound head

biopsy needle

lymph nodes

may be used to remove a larger sample. The needle is often guided into the tumor with imaging. When mammography is used during a biopsy, it is called a stereotactic needle biopsy.

One or more clips may be placed near the breast tumor during a biopsy. The clips are small, painless, and made of metal. They will mark the site for future treatment and imaging. The clips stay in place until surgery. If the area biopsied is benign, the clip will remain in place to mark the biopsy site on future imaging.

There are both physical and emotional experiences in having biopsies. You may need to rest and place an ice pack on the biopsy area after the procedure. If you are working or have other commitments, you may want to take the day off to recover emotionally and physically from the experience.

Axillary lymph node needle biopsy

An axillary lymph node (ALN) drains lymph fluid from the breast and nearby areas. In an axillary lymph node biopsy, a sample of lymph node near the armpit (axilla) is biopsied with a needle. This is to determine if abnormal lymph nodes seen on imaging tests contain cancer cells. An ultrasound-guided fine-needle aspiration (US-FNA) or core biopsy will be used. If cancer is found, it is called node positive (node+). A marker may be placed in the node so that it can be identified later if needed.

Create a medical binder

A medical binder or notebook is a great way to organize all of your records in one place.

- Make copies of blood tests, imaging results, and reports about your specific type of cancer. It will be helpful when getting a second opinion.

- Choose a binder that meets your needs. Consider a zipper pocket to include a pen, small calendar, and insurance cards.

- Create folders for insurance forms, medical records, and tests results. You can do the same on your computer.

- Use online patient portals to view your test results and other records. Download or print the records to add to your binder.

- Organize your binder in a way that works for you. Add a section for questions and to take notes.

- Bring your medical binder to appointments. You never know when you might need it!

Hormone receptor status

A hormone is a substance made by a gland in your body. Your blood carries hormones throughout your body. A receptor is a protein found inside or on the surface of a cell such as a cancer cell. Substances such as hormones attach (bind) to these receptors. This causes changes within the cell.

Hormones recognize and bind to specific hormone receptors.

There are 2 types of hormone receptors:

> **Estrogen** – plays a role in breast development

> **Progesterone** – plays a role in menstrual cycle and pregnancy

Once these hormones attach to receptors inside breast cancer cells, they can cause cancer to grow. If found, these receptors may be targeted using endocrine therapy.

Immunohistochemistry

Immunohistochemistry (IHC) is a special staining process that involves adding a chemical marker to cells. These cells are then studied using a microscope. IHC can find estrogen and progesterone receptors in breast cancer cells. A pathologist will measure how many cells have estrogen and/or progesterone receptors and the number of receptors inside each cell.

Hormone receptor-positive

In hormone receptor-positive (HR+) breast cancer, IHC finds estrogen and/or progesterone hormone receptors. Most breast cancers are HR+.

There are 2 types of HR+ cells:

> **Estrogen receptor-positive (ER+)** cancer cells may need estrogen to grow. These cells may stop growing or die with treatment to block estrogen production or estrogen receptor signaling.

> **Progesterone receptor-positive (PR+)** cancer cells need progesterone to grow.

Hormone receptor-positive breast cancer is treated with endocrine therapy.

Hormone receptor-negative

Hormone receptor-negative (HR-) breast cancer cells do not have either estrogen or progesterone hormone receptors. These cancers are sometimes simply called hormone negative. HR- cancers often grow faster than hormone receptor-positive cancers. Both the estrogen and progesterone receptors need to be negative for the cancer to be considered HR-.

There are 2 types of HR- cells:

> **Estrogen receptor-negative (ER-)** cancer cells do not have an estrogen receptor. These cancer cells do not need estrogen to grow and continue to grow despite treatment to block estrogen.

> **Progesterone receptor-negative (PR-)** cancer cells do not need progesterone to grow.

HER2 status

Human epidermal growth factor receptor 2 (HER2) is a protein involved in normal cell growth. It is found on the surface of all cells. When amounts are high, it causes cells to grow and divide. Some breast cancers have too many HER2 genes or receptors. Too many HER2s is called HER2-positive (HER2+). You might hear it called HER2 overexpression or amplification.

There are 2 tests for HER2:

> **Immunohistochemistry (IHC)** measures receptors. If the IHC score is 3+, the cancer is HER2+. If the score is 0 or 1, it is considered HER2-. If the score is 2+, further testing is needed.

> **In situ hybridization (ISH)** counts the number of copies of the HER2 gene. This test is done mainly when the IHC score is unclear.

You might have more than one HER2 test. HER2 tests are done using a tumor biopsy sample.

Biomarker testing

A sample from a biopsy of your tumor may be tested to look for specific DNA (deoxyribonucleic acid) mutations/alterations, protein levels, or other molecular features. This information is used to choose the best treatment for you. It is sometimes called molecular testing or tumor profiling.

Biomarker testing includes tests of genes or their products (proteins). It identifies the presence or absence of mutations and certain proteins that might suggest treatment. Proteins are written like this: BRCA. Genes are written with italics like this: *BRCA*. HER2 and hormone receptor status are part of biomarker testing. Not all of the tests listed below are done for all patients. Your treatment team will recommend the best types of biomarker testing that are important for you.

Tumor markers

Your blood or biopsy tissue may be tested for proteins. These proteins are called tumor markers. Knowing this information can help plan treatment. Examples of some tumor markers in breast cancer include carcinoembryonic antigen (CEA), CA 15-3, and CA 27.29. An increase in the level of certain tumor markers could mean that the cancer has grown or spread (progressed). However, not everyone has elevated levels of these markers and tumor markers alone are not a reliable method of detecting breast cancer.

Tumor mutation burden

When there are 10 or more mutations per million base pairs of tumor DNA, it is called tumor mutational burden-high (TMB-H). TMB-H can be used to help predict response to cancer treatment using immune checkpoint inhibitors that target the proteins called programmed death protein 1 (PD-1) and programmed death-ligand 1 (PD-L1).

Tumor mutation testing

A sample of your tumor or blood may be used to see if the cancer cells have any specific DNA mutations. This is a different type of DNA testing than the genetic testing for mutations you may have inherited from your parents. In tumor mutation testing, only the tumor is tested and not the rest of your body. Certain mutations such as PIK3CA can be targeted with specific therapies.

MSI-H/dMMR

Microsatellites are short, repeated strings of DNA. When errors or defects occur, they are fixed by mismatch repair (MMR) proteins. Some cancers prevent these errors from being fixed. This is called microsatellite instability (MSI) or deficient mismatch repair (dMMR). When cancer cells have more than a normal number of microsatellites, it is called microsatellite instability-high (MSI-H). This is often due to dMMR genes.

PD-1 and PD-L1 testing

Programmed death protein 1 (PD-1) and programmed death-ligand 1 (PD-L1) are immune proteins. If either protein is expressed on the surface of cancer cells, it can cause your immune cells to ignore the cancer and suppress the anti-tumor immune response. If your cancer expresses either protein, you might have treatment that combines chemotherapy and a checkpoint inhibitor therapy. This is designed to activate your immune system to better fight off the cancer cells.

FISH

Fluorescence in situ hybridization (FISH) is a testing method that involves special dyes called probes that attach to pieces of DNA, the genetic material in a person's cells.

Immunohistochemistry

Immunohistochemistry (IHC) is a special staining process that involves adding a chemical marker to cancer or immune cells. The cells are then studied using a microscope.

Next-generation sequencing

Next-generation sequencing (NGS) is a high-throughput method used to determine a portion of a person's DNA sequence. This method would only be used if enough tumor tissue remains after other biomarker testing has been completed.

PCR

A polymerase chain reaction (PCR) is a lab process that can make millions or billions of copies of your DNA (genetic information). PCR is very sensitive. It can find 1 abnormal cell among more than 100,000 normal cells. These copies called PCR product might be used for NGS.

Genetic risk testing

About 1 out of 10 breast cancers are hereditary. Depending on your family history or other features of your cancer, your health care provider might refer you for genetic testing to learn more about your cancer. A genetic counselor or trained provider will speak to you about the results. Tests results may be used to guide treatment planning.

Genetic testing is done using blood or saliva (spitting into a cup). The goal is to look for gene mutations inherited from your biological parents called germline mutations. Some mutations can put you at risk for more than one type of cancer. You can pass these genes on to your children. Also, family members might carry these mutations. Tell your doctor if there is a family history of cancer.

BRCA tests

Everyone has *BRCA* genes. Normal *BRCA* genes help to prevent tumor growth. They help fix damaged cells and help cells grow normally. *BRCA* mutations are *BRCA* genes that are not functioning normally, thereby putting you at risk for developing multiple types of cancer. Mutations in *BRCA1* or *BRCA2* increase the risk of breast, ovarian, prostate, colorectal, pancreatic, and melanoma skin cancers. Mutated *BRCA* genes can also affect how well some treatments work.

What is your family health history?

Some cancers and other diseases run in families – those who are related to you through genes passed down from parent to child. This information is called a family health history. You can ask family members about their health issues like heart disease, cancer, and diabetes, and at what age they were diagnosed. For relatives who have died, ask about the cause and age of death.

Start by asking your parents, siblings, and children. Next, talk to half-siblings, aunts and uncles, niece and nephews, grandparents, and grandchildren.

Write down what you learn about your family history and share with your health care provider.

Some of the questions to ask include:

- Do you have any chronic diseases, such as heart disease or diabetes, or health conditions such as high blood pressure or high cholesterol?

- Have you had any other diseases, such as cancer or stroke?

- How old were you when each of these diseases and health conditions was diagnosed?

- What is our family's ancestry – from what countries did our ancestors originate?

Distress screening

It is normal to have strong feelings about being diagnosed with cancer and your feelings can also change from day-to-day and week-to-week. Talk to your doctor and with those whom you feel most comfortable about how you are feeling. There are services and people who can help you. Support and counseling are available. Dealing with a cancer diagnosis may sometimes be stressful and may cause distress. Your treatment team will screen your level of distress. This is part of your cancer care.

Distress is an unpleasant experience of a mental, physical, social, or spiritual nature. It can affect how you feel, think, and act. Distress might include feelings of sadness, fear, helplessness, worry, anger, and guilt. You may also experience depression, anxiety, and sleeping problems.

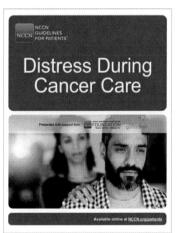

For more information, read the *NCCN Guidelines for Patients: Distress During Cancer Care*, available at <u>NCCN. org/patientguidelines</u>.

Performance status

Performance status (PS) is a person's general level of fitness and ability to perform daily tasks. Your state of general health will be rated using a PS scale called ECOG (Eastern Cooperative Oncology Group) or the Karnofsky Performance Status (KPS). Your performance status can help to determine your ability to tolerate treatments such as surgery or chemotherapy.

ECOG PS
The ECOG PS scores range from 0 to 4.

> ➤ PS 0 means you are fully active.

> ➤ PS 1 means you are still able to perform light to moderate activity.

> ➤ PS 2 means you can still care for yourself but are not active.

> ➤ PS 3 means you are limited to the chair or bed more than half of the time.

> ➤ PS 4 means you need someone to care for you and are limited to a chair or bed.

In breast cancer, PS might be referred to as good or poor. Good PS is usually PS 0 or PS 1.

Karnofsky PS
The KPS score ranges from 0 to 100.

> ➤ 10 to 40 means you cannot care for yourself without the help of others.

> ➤ 50 to 70 means you cannot work and need some help to take care of yourself.

> ➤ 80 to 100 means you are completely independent and can carry out daily tasks.

Key points

- Tests are used to find cancer, plan treatment, and check how well treatment is working.

- You will have a physical exam, including a breast exam, to see if anything feels or looks abnormal.

- Treatment can affect your fertility, the ability to have children.

- Blood tests check for signs of disease and how well organs are working.

- Imaging tests take pictures of the inside of your body.

- A bilateral diagnostic mammogram includes detailed pictures of both breasts. It is different than a screening mammogram.

- During a biopsy, tissue or fluid samples are removed for testing. Samples are needed to confirm the presence of cancer and to perform cancer cell tests.

- A sample from a biopsy of your tumor will be tested for estrogen receptor (ER) status, progesterone receptor (PR) status, HER2 status, and grade (histology). This can tell doctors about the behavior of your cancer, as well as treatments your cancer may respond to.

- About 1 out of 10 breast cancers are hereditary. Depending on your family history or other features of your cancer, your might be referred for genetic testing, to speak with a genetic counselor, and possibly have genetic testing.

- Online portals are a great way to access your test results.

> Testing takes time. It might take days or weeks for all test results to come in.

3
Breast cancer staging

26　Overview

28　Stages

30　Key points

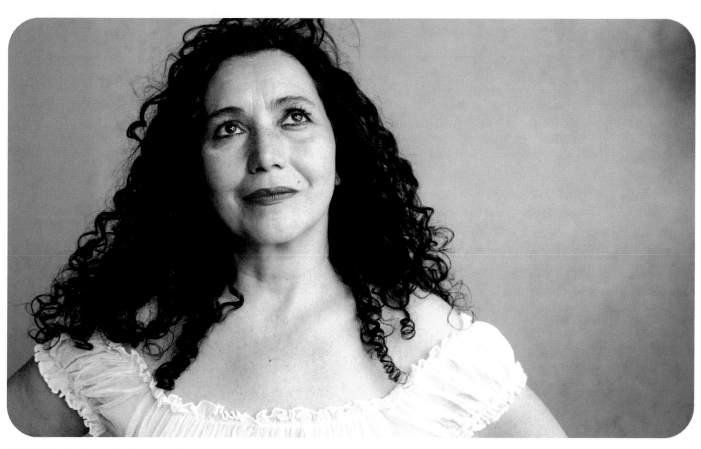

Cancer staging is used to make treatment decisions. It describes the size and location of the tumor and if cancer has spread to lymph nodes, organs, or other parts of the body. This chapter explains invasive breast cancer stages.

Overview

Breast cancer staging is often done twice, before and after surgery. Staging after surgery provides more specific details about the size of the cancer and lymph node status.

> **Clinical stage (c)** is the rating given before any treatment. It is based on a physical exam, biopsy, and imaging tests. An example might look like cN2 or cM1.

> **Pathologic stage (p)** or surgical stage is determined by examining tissue removed during surgery. An example might be pN2. If you are given drug therapy before surgery, then the stage might look like ypT3.

A cancer stage is a way to describe the extent of the cancer at the time you are first diagnosed. The American Joint Committee on Cancer (AJCC) created a staging system to determine how much cancer is in your body, where it is located, and what subtype you have. This is called staging. Based on testing, your cancer will be assigned a stage. Staging helps to predict prognosis and is needed to make treatment decisions. AJCC is just one type of staging system.

Staging is based on a combination of information to reach a final numbered stage. Often, not all information is available at the initial evaluation. More information can be gathered as treatment begins. Doctors may explain your cancer stage in different ways than described next.

Information gathered during staging:

> **The extent (size) of the tumor (T)**: How large is the cancer? Has it grown into nearby areas?

> **The spread to nearby lymph nodes (N)**: Has the cancer spread to nearby lymph nodes? If so, how many? Where?

> **The spread (metastasis) to distant sites (M)**: Has the cancer spread to distant organs such as the lungs or liver?

> **Estrogen receptor (ER) status:** Does the cancer have the protein called an estrogen receptor?

> **Progesterone receptor (PR) status**: Does the cancer have the protein called a progesterone receptor?

> **Human epidermal growth factor receptor 2 (HER2) status**: Does the cancer make too much of a protein called HER2?

> **Grade of the cancer (G)**: How much do the cancer cells look like normal cells?

TNM scores

The tumor, node, metastasis (TNM) system is used to stage breast cancer. In this system, the letters T, N, and M describe different areas of cancer growth. Based on cancer test results, your doctor will assign a score or number to each letter. The higher the number, the larger the tumor or the more the cancer has spread. These scores will be combined to assign the cancer a stage. A TNM example might look like this: T1N0M0 or T1, N0, M0.

> **T (tumor)** – Depth and spread of the main (primary) tumor(s) in one or both breasts

> **N (node)** – If cancer has spread to nearby (regional) lymph nodes

> **M (metastasis)** – If cancer has spread to distant parts of the body or metastasized

Grade

Grade describes how abnormal the tumor cells look under a microscope (called histology). Higher-grade cancers tend to grow and spread faster than lower-grade cancers. GX means the grade can't be determined, followed by G1, G2, and G3. G3 is the highest grade for breast cancers. A low-grade tumor has a lower risk of recurrence. A high-grade tumor has a higher risk for recurrence (of cancer returning).

> **GX** – Grade cannot be determined

> **G1** – Low grade

> **G2** – Intermediate grade

> **G3** – High grade

Numbered stages

Numbered stages are based on TNM scores. Stages range from stage 0 to stage 4, with 4 being the most advanced. Doctors write these stages as stage I, stage II, stage III, and stage IV. For example, ductal carcinoma in situ (DCIS) is stage 0 or Tis, N0, M0.

Stage 0 is noninvasive

Noninvasive breast cancer is rated stage 0. DCIS is found only in the ducts (Tis). It has not spread to the surrounding breast tissue, lymph nodes (N0), or distant sites (M0).

For more information on DCIS, read the *NCCN Guidelines for Patients: Breast Cancer – Ductal Carcinoma In Situ,* available at NCCN. org/patientguidelines.

Stages 1, 2, and 3 are invasive

Invasive breast cancer is rated stage 1, 2, or 3. It has grown outside the ducts, lobules, or breast skin. Cancer might be in the axillary lymph nodes.

Stage 4 is metastatic

In stage 4 breast cancer, cancer has spread to distant sites (M1), but can also be found in the axillary lymph nodes. Your first diagnosis can be stage 4 metastatic breast cancer (called de novo) or it can develop from earlier stages.

For more information on metastatic breast cancer, read the *NCCN Guidelines for Patients: Breast Cancer – Metastatic,* available at NCCN.org/patientguidelines.

Stages

Staging of invasive breast cancer is complex. It takes into account what can be felt during a physical exam, what can be seen on imaging tests, and what is found during a biopsy or surgery. Keep copies of your pathology reports. The pathology report might include a lot of abbreviations such as pN0(mol+), ypT2, or cN3. Your doctor can help explain what they mean.

The following section describes general clinical staging of invasive breast cancer. These stages can be found in Guide 2.

T = Tumor

The primary tumor size can be measured in centimeters (cm) or millimeters (mm). One inch is equal to 2.54 cm. A large pea is 1 cm (10 mm). A golf ball is 4 cm (40 mm). A tumor micrometastasis is a very small cancerous cell that is smaller than 1 mm. It might be written as T1mi. Ipsilateral means on the same side of the body.

- > **T1 Tumor** is 2 cm (20 mm) or less

  - **T1mi Tumor** is micrometastasis of 1 mm or less

  - **T1a Tumor** is 1.1 mm to 5 mm

  - **T1b Tumor** is 5.1 mm to 10 mm

  - **T1c Tumor** is 10.1 mm to 20 mm

- > **T2 Tumor** is 2.1 cm to 5 cm

- > **T3 Tumor** is more than 5 cm

- > **T4 Tumor** is of any size and has invaded nearby structures such the chest wall and skin of the breast

- > **T4d** Inflammatory carcinoma

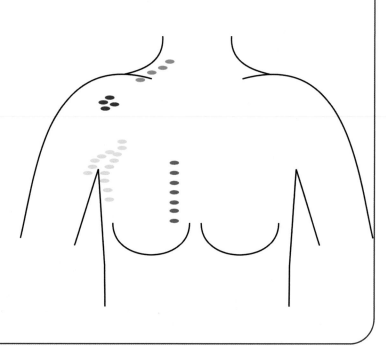

Clinical staging

Clinical staging of lymph nodes is staging before surgery.

- ◯ **Cancer is in axillary nodes**
- ⬤ **Cancer is in internal mammary nodes**
- ⬤ **Cancer is in infraclavicular nodes**
- ⬤ **Cancer is in supraclavicular nodes**

N = Regional lymph node

There are hundreds of lymph nodes throughout your body. They work as filters to help fight infection and remove harmful things from your body. Regional lymph nodes are those located near the tumor in the breast. If breast cancer spreads, it often goes first to nearby lymph nodes under the arm. It can also sometimes spread to lymph nodes near the collarbone or near the breast bone. Knowing if the cancer has spread to your lymph nodes helps doctors find the best way to treat your cancer.

> **N0** means no cancer is in the regional lymph nodes. Isolated tumor cells (ITCs) may be present. These are malignant cell clusters no larger than 0.2 mm.

> **N1mi** means micrometastases (approximately 200 cells, larger than 0.2 mm, but none larger than 2.0 mm) are found in lymph nodes.

> **N1, N2, N3** means regional lymph node metastases are found. The higher the number, the more lymph nodes that have metastases.

M = Metastasis

Cancer that has spread to distant parts of the body is shown as M1. This is metastatic breast cancer (MBC). The most common sites for metastasis are bone and lung.

> **M0** means no known distant metastasis.

> **M1** means distant metastasis is found. This is metastatic breast cancer.

Guide 2 Invasive breast cancer: Stage 1A through 3C	
Stage 0	• Tis, N0, M0 ductal carcinoma in situ (DCIS)
Stage 1A	• T1, N0, M0
Stage 1B	• T0, N1mi, M0 • T1, N1mi, M0
Stage 2A	• T0, N1, M0 • T1, N1, M0 • T2, N0, M0
Stage 2B	• T2, N1, M0 • T3, N0, M0
Stage 3A	• T0, N2, M0 • T1, N2, M0 • T2, N2, M0 • T3, N1, M0 • T3, N2, M0
Stage 3B	• T4, N0, M0 • T4, N1, M0 • T4, N2, M0
Stage 3C	• Any T, N3, M0
Stage 4	• Any T, Any N, M1 metastatic breast cancer (MBC)

Key points

- › Staging is used to make treatment decisions.

- › Doctors rate the extent of breast cancer in the body using the tumor, node, metastasis (TNM) system.

- › Breast cancer is often staged twice, before and after surgery.

- › Clinical stage (c) is the rating given before any treatment. It is written as cTNM.

- › The pathologic stage (p) is based on the results of tissue removed during surgery. It is written as pTNM.

- › Grade describes how abnormal the tumor cells look under a microscope (called histology).

- › Regional lymph nodes are found near the breast.

- › Doctors may explain your cancer stage in different ways to make it less confusing.

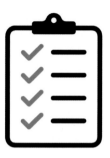

We want your feedback!

Our goal is to provide helpful and easy-to-understand information on cancer.

Take our survey to let us know what we got right and what we could do better:

NCCN.org/patients/feedback

4
Treatment overview

32	Treatment team
34	Overview
34	Surgery
39	Radiation therapy
40	Chemotherapy
41	HER2-targeted therapy
41	Endocrine therapy
44	Bone-strengthening therapy
45	Inhibitors

45	Immunotherapy
46	Clinical trials
48	Supportive care
51	Key points

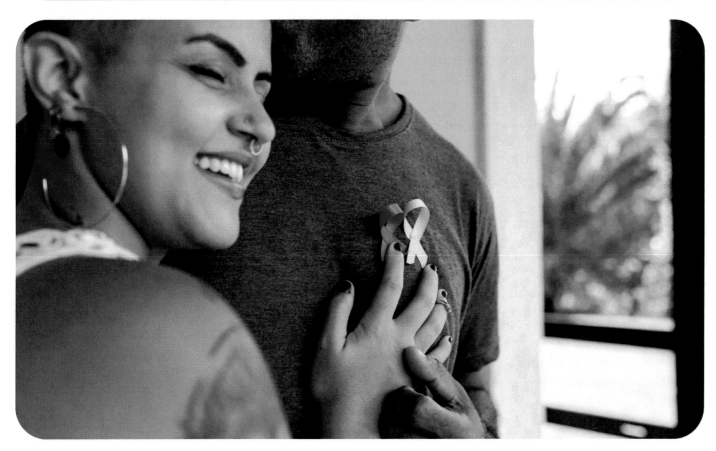

There is more than one treatment for invasive breast cancer. This chapter describes treatment options and what to expect. Together, you and your doctor will choose a treatment plan that is best for you.

Treatment team

Treating breast cancer takes a team approach. Treatment decisions should involve a multidisciplinary team (MDT). An MDT is a team of doctors, health care workers, and social care professionals from different professional backgrounds who have knowledge (expertise) and experience with your type of cancer. This team is united in the planning and implementing of your treatment. Ask who will coordinate your care.

Some members of your care team will be with you throughout cancer treatment, while others will only be there for parts of it. Get to know your care team and help them get to know you.

Depending on your diagnosis, your team might include the following:

> **A pathologist** analyzes the cells, tissues, and organs removed during a biopsy or surgery and provides cancer diagnosis, staging, and information about biomarker testing.

> **A diagnostic radiologist** interprets the results of mammograms, MRIs, and other imaging tests.

> **An interventional radiologist** performs needle biopsies and places ports for treatment.

> **A surgical oncologist** performs operations to remove cancer.

> **A reconstructive (plastic) surgeon** performs breast reconstruction, if desired, for those who undergo mastectomy.

> **A medical oncologist** treats cancer in adults using systemic therapy such as endocrine or targeted therapy.

> **A radiation oncologist** prescribes and plans radiation therapy to treat cancer.

> **An anesthesiologist** gives anesthesia, a medicine so you do not feel pain during surgery or procedures.

> **Residents and fellows** are doctors who are continuing their training, some to become specialists in a certain field of medicine.

> **Nurse practitioners and physician assistants** are health care providers who work alongside doctors and other members of the medical team. Some of your clinic visits may be done by a nurse practitioner or physician assistant.

> **Oncology nurses** provide your hands-on care, like giving systemic therapy, managing your care, answering questions, and helping you cope with side effects. Sometimes, these experts are called nurse navigators.

> **Oncology pharmacists** provide medicines used to treat cancer and to manage symptoms and side effects.

> **Palliative care nurses, advanced practice providers**, **and physicians** help provide an extra layer of support with your cancer-related symptoms.

> **Nutritionists and dietitians** can provide guidance on what foods are most suitable for your condition.

> **An occupational therapist** helps people with the tasks of daily living.

> **A physical therapist** helps people move with greater comfort and ease.

> **A certified lymphedema therapist** gives a type of massage called manual lymph drainage.

> **Psychologists and psychiatrists** are mental health experts who can help manage issues such as depression, anxiety, or other mental health conditions that can affect how you feel.

> **Social workers** help people solve and cope with problems in their everyday lives. Clinical social workers also diagnose and treat mental, behavioral, and emotional issues. The anxiety a person feels when diagnosed with cancer might be managed by a social worker in some cancer centers.

> **A research team** helps to collect research data and coordinate care if you are in a clinical trial.

Your physical, mental, and emotional well-being are important. You know yourself better than anyone. Help other team members understand:

> How you feel

> What you need

> What is working and what is not

Keep a list of names and contact information for each member of your team. This will make

If you smoke or vape

If you smoke tobacco or use e-cigarettes, it is very important to quit. Smoking can limit how well cancer treatment works. Smoking greatly increases your chances of having side effects during and after surgery, including breast reconstruction. It also increases your chances of developing other cancers.

Nicotine is the chemical in tobacco that makes you want to keep smoking. Nicotine withdrawal is challenging for most smokers. The stress of having cancer may make it even harder to quit. If you smoke, ask your doctor about counseling and medicines to help you quit.

For online support, try these websites:

* SmokeFree.gov

* BeTobaccoFree.gov

* CDC.gov/tobacco

it easier for you and anyone involved in your care to know whom to contact with questions or concerns.

Overview

Invasive breast cancer is treatable. Treatment can be local, systemic, or usually a combination of both. It is important to have regular talks with your doctor about your goals for treatment and your treatment plan.

There are 2 types of treatment:

> **Local therapy** focuses on the breast and lymph node area. It includes surgery, ablation, and radiation therapy.

> **Systemic therapy** works throughout the body. It includes endocrine therapy, chemotherapy, and targeted therapy.

There are many treatment options. However, not everyone will respond to treatment in the same way. Some people will do better than expected. Others will do worse. Many factors play a role in how you will respond to treatment.

Birth control during treatment

If you become pregnant during chemotherapy, radiation therapy, endocrine therapy, or other types of systemic therapy, serious birth defects can occur. If you had menstrual periods before starting chemotherapy, use birth control without hormones. Condoms are an option. "The pill" or other types of hormonal birth control are usually not recommended, especially in hormone receptor-positive cancers. Speak to your doctor about preventing pregnancy while being treated for breast cancer.

Those who want to become pregnant in the future should be referred to a fertility specialist to discuss options before starting chemotherapy and/or endocrine therapy.

Surgery

Surgery is an operation or procedure to remove cancer from the body. Surgery is the main or primary treatment for invasive breast cancer. This is only one part of a treatment plan. Systemic therapy or radiation therapy might be used before surgery to shrink the tumor or reduce the amount of cancer (called cancer burden).

> **Preoperative** is treatment before surgery. It also called neoadjuvant therapy.

> **Postoperative** is treatment after surgery. It is also called adjuvant therapy.

When preparing for surgery, seek the opinion of an experienced surgeon. The surgeon should be an expert in performing your type of surgery. Hospitals that perform many surgeries often have better results. You can ask for a referral to a hospital or cancer center that has experience in treating your type of cancer.

The removal of the cancer through surgery can be accomplished in different ways depending on the specific circumstances, such as the size and location of the tumor, and if there is cancer in any surrounding organs and tissues.

Surgery might be a lumpectomy or mastectomy. It is based on the safest and best way to remove the cancer. If you are considering breast reconstruction, surgery requires collaboration between a breast surgeon and the reconstructive (plastic) surgeon. Surgery usually includes removal of some lymph nodes.

Goal of surgery

The goal of surgery or tumor resection is to remove all of the cancer and obtain tissue for pathologic staging. To do so, the tumor is removed along with some normal-looking tissue around its edge called the surgical margin. The surgical margin may look normal, but cancerous cells may be found when viewed under a microscope by a pathologist. A clear or negative margin (R0) is when no cancer cells are found in the tissue around the edge of the tumor. In a positive margin, cancer cells are found in normal-looking tissue around the tumor. The lymph nodes are also checked, either with a sentinel lymph node biopsy or axillary lymph node dissection.

Surgical margins

The goal of surgery is a cancer-free surgical margin. After surgery, you will likely receive treatment such as systemic therapy and/or radiation to kill any remaining cancer cells in the area.

> **In a clear or negative margin (R0),** no cancerous cells are found in the tissue around the edge of the tumor.

> **In an R1 positive margin,** the surgeon removes all the visible tumor, but the microscopic margins are still positive for tumor cells. Despite best efforts this can happen.

> **In an R2 positive margin,** the surgeon is unable to remove all the visible tumor or there is metastatic disease.

A negative margin (R0) is the best result. Your surgeon will look carefully for cancer not only along the surgical margin, but in other nearby areas. Despite best efforts, it is not always possible to find all of the cancer. Sometimes, surgeons can't safely remove the tumor with a cancer-free margin.

You might have more than one surgery. You might also have a wound drain to prevent fluid from collecting in the body after surgery. These drains are usually removed a few days after surgery.

Lumpectomy

Lumpectomy is the removal of the abnormal cells or tumor in the breast. It is also called breast-conserving therapy or breast-conserving surgery (BCS). In a lumpectomy, only the tumor with an area of normal tissue will be removed. The rest of your breast is left alone. Extra tissue is removed around the tumor to create a cancer-free area. This cancer-free area is called a surgical margin. Having a surgical margin will decrease the chance that cancer may return in that area of the breast. You may have more than one surgery to ensure all of the cancer was removed.

The breast might not look the same after a lumpectomy. Speak to your doctor about how a lumpectomy might affect the look and shape of your breast, and any concerns you have. Certain reconstruction options, such as volume displacement, might be available.

Mastectomy

In a mastectomy, all of the breast tissue underneath the skin is removed. The nipple, lymph nodes, and muscle might be removed as well. Before removing the breast, the surgeon may do a sentinel lymph node biopsy (SLNB). Sentinel lymph nodes are the first nodes cancer cells are likely to have spread from the main tumor.

Types of mastectomy include:

> **A total mastectomy** or simple mastectomy is a surgery that removes the whole breast with a flat skin closure. Chest muscle is not removed.

> **A skin-sparing mastectomy** removes the breast but not all of the skin, in order to have breast reconstruction that might include flaps and/or implants.

> **Nipple-sparing mastectomy** preserves the nipple areola complex (NAC) as well. Not everyone is a candidate for nipple-sparing mastectomy.

Breast reconstruction is an option after a mastectomy. It might be done at the same time as mastectomy ("immediate") or at some time following the completion of cancer treatment ("delayed"). Breast reconstruction is often done in stages.

Sentinel lymph node biopsy

Sentinel lymph nodes (SLNs) are the first lymph nodes that cancer cells are most likely to spread to from a primary tumor. Sometimes, there is only one sentinel lymph node, but usually there is more than one. A sentinel lymph node biopsy (SLNB or SNB) is done during surgery such as a mastectomy or lumpectomy to determine if any cancer cells have traveled to the lymph nodes. The lymph nodes removed are called the sentinel nodes. They may or may not contain any cancer cells. Just because these nodes are removed, it does not mean that they are positive for cancer.

To find the sentinel lymph nodes, a radioactive material and other dyes are injected into the breast where they travel through the lymphatics in the breast to the lymph nodes. This helps the surgeon find which of the nodes are the sentinel lymph nodes. Once the nodes are found, they are removed and tested by a pathologist. If cancer is found, all of the lymph nodes may need to be removed. This is called axillary lymph node dissection.

Axillary lymph node dissection

An axillary lymph node dissection (ALND) is surgery to remove all of the axillary lymph nodes. This is performed after an axillary lymph node biopsy or SLNB shows cancer in the lymph nodes (called node positive). Then, an ALND will remove any other lymph nodes that contain cancer. Removing lymph nodes can cause lymphedema and other health issues.

If the axillary nodes are removed along with the breast, it is called a modified radical mastectomy.

There are 3 levels of axillary lymph nodes:

- ➤ **Level I** – nodes located below the lower edge of the chest muscle

- ➤ **Level II** – nodes located underneath the chest muscle

- ➤ **Level III** – nodes located above the chest muscle near the collarbone

An ALND usually removes level I and II axillary lymph nodes. For more information about the timing of biopsies, talk with your care team.

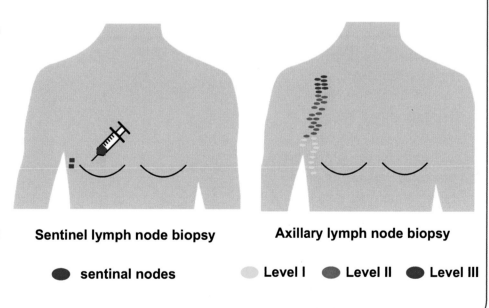

Lymph node surgery

There are two types of surgeries to remove lymph nodes. A sentinel lymph node biopsy finds and removes the lymph nodes where breast cancer first spreads. An axillary lymph node dissection removes lymph nodes from levels I and II.

Sentinel lymph node biopsy

● sentinal nodes

Axillary lymph node biopsy

○ Level I   ● Level II   ● Level III

Total (simple) mastectomy

The dotted line shows where the entire breast is removed. Some lymph nodes under the arm may also be removed

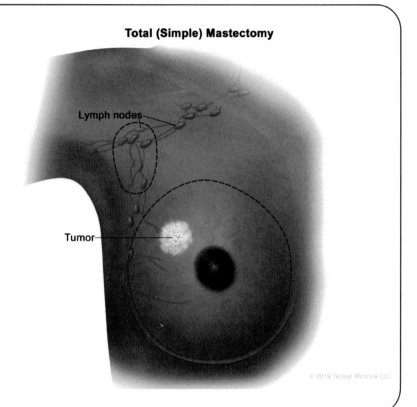

Total (Simple) Mastectomy

Lymph nodes

Tumor

© 2019 Terese Winslow LLC

Modified radical mastectomy

The dotted line shows where the entire breast and some lymph nodes are removed. Part of the chest wall muscle may also be removed.

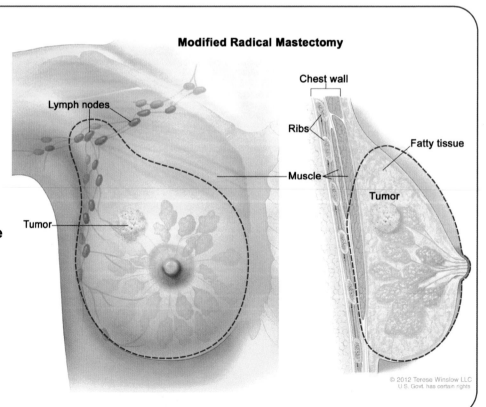

Modified Radical Mastectomy

Lymph nodes

Tumor

Chest wall

Ribs

Fatty tissue

Muscle

Tumor

© 2012 Terese Winslow LLC
U.S. Govt. has certain rights

Radiation therapy

Radiation therapy (RT) uses high-energy radiation from x-rays, photons, protons, electrons, and other sources to kill cancer cells and shrink tumors. It is given over a certain period of time. Radiation therapy can be given alone or before or after surgery to treat or slow the growth of cancer. Sometimes, radiation is given with certain systemic therapies. It may be used as supportive care to help ease pain or discomfort caused by cancer.

Types of radiation therapy:

> **Whole breast radiation therapy (WBRT)** is used to treat the whole breast. Sometimes, additional treatments may be given to the tumor area. This is called a "boost."

> **Accelerated partial breast irradiation (APBI)** is used to treat only the area where the tumor was removed.

> **Lymph node radiation therapy** is used to treat the area of lymph nodes. It is also called regional nodal irradiation (RNI).

Radiation may be given to the breast and chest wall, infraclavicular region (below the collarbone), supraclavicular area (above the collarbone), lymph nodes found inside the breast (internal mammary), or axillary bed (armpit).

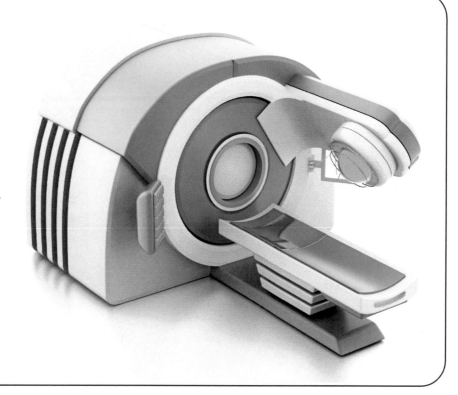

Radiation therapy

Radiation therapy uses high-energy radiation from x-rays, gamma rays, protons, and other sources to kill cancer cells and shrink tumors. It is also used to treat pain caused by cancer.

Chemotherapy

Chemotherapy kills fast-growing cells throughout the body, including cancer cells and some normal cells. More than one chemotherapy may be used to treat invasive breast cancer. When only one drug is used, it's called a single agent. A combination or multi-agent regimen is the use of two or more chemotherapy drugs.

Some chemotherapy drugs are liquids that are infused into a vein or injected under the skin with a needle. Other chemotherapy drugs may be given as a pill that is swallowed.

Some examples of chemotherapy drugs include:

- Capecitabine (Xeloda)
- Carboplatin
- Cisplatin (Platinol)
- Cyclophosphamide
- Docetaxel (Taxotere)
- Doxorubicin (Adriamycin, Rubex)
- Doxorubicin liposomal injection (Doxil)
- Epirubicin (Ellence)
- Eribulin (Halaven)
- Fluorouracil
- Gemcitabine (Gemzar, Infugem)
- Methotrexate
- Ixabepilone (Ixempra Kit)
- Paclitaxel (Taxol, Abraxane)
- Vinorelbine (Navelbine)

Doxorubicin, doxorubicin liposomal injection (Doxil), and epirubicin (Ellence) are also called anthracyclines.

Docetaxel, paclitaxel, and albumin-bound paclitaxel are also called taxanes.

Capecitabine (Xeloda), fluorouracil, gemcitabine (Gemzar, Infugem), and methotrexate are also called anti-metabolites.

Most chemotherapy is given in cycles of treatment days followed by days of rest. This allows the body to recover before the next cycle. Cycles vary in length depending on which drugs are used. The number of treatment days per cycle and the total number of cycles given also varies.

Myeloid growth factors

Certain chemotherapies can reduce the cells that fight infection. Treatments with myeloid growth factors (MGFs) can help increase the number of blood cells and prevent infections.

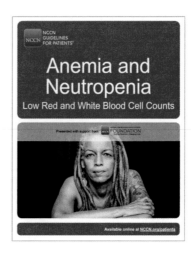

For more information on myeloid growth factors, see *NCCN Guidelines for Patients: Anemia and Neutropenia*, available at NCCN.org/patientguidelines.

HER2-targeted therapy

HER2 is a protein involved in normal cell growth. There might be higher amounts of HER2 in your breast cancer. If this is the case, it is called HER2-positive (HER2+) breast cancer. HER2-targeted therapy is drug therapy that treats HER2+ breast cancer. Most often, HER2-targeted therapy is given with chemotherapy. However, it might be used alone or in combination with endocrine therapy.

HER2-targeted therapies include:

> Pertuzumab (Perjeta)

> Trastuzumab (Herceptin) or trastuzumab substitutes (biosimilars) such as Kanjinti, Ogivri, Herzuma, Ontruzant, and Trazimera

> Ado-trastuzumab emtansine (T-DM1) (Kadcyla)

> Fam-trastuzumab deruxtecan-nxki (Enhertu)

> Lapatinib (Tykerb)

> Margetuximab-cmkb (Margenza)

> Neratinib (Nerlynx)

> Tucatinib (Tukysa)

> Phesgo as a substitute for combination therapy of trastuzumab with pertuzumab

Your heart will be monitored before and during treatment with trastuzumab. Tests will measure the left ventricular ejection fraction (LVEF), the amount of blood pumping from the left side of the heart.

> You should not become pregnant during treatment with radiation therapy or systemic therapy.

Endocrine therapy

Endocrine therapy blocks estrogen or progesterone to treat hormone receptor-positive (HR+) breast cancer. The endocrine system is made up of organs and tissues that produce hormones. Hormones are natural chemicals released into the bloodstream.

There are 4 hormones that might be targeted in endocrine therapy:

> **Estrogen** is made mainly by the ovaries.

> **Progesterone** is made mainly by the ovaries.

> **Luteinizing hormone-releasing hormone (LHRH)** is made by a part of the brain called the hypothalamus. It tells the ovaries to make estrogen and progesterone and testicles to make testosterone. LHRH is also called gonadotropin-releasing hormone (GnRH).

> **Androgen** is made by the adrenal glands, testicles, and ovaries.

Hormones can cause breast cancer to grow. Endocrine therapy will stop your body from making hormones or it will block what hormones do in the body. This can slow tumor growth or shrink the tumor for a period of time.

Endocrine therapy is sometimes called hormone therapy. It is not the same as hormone replacement therapy used for menopause.

More than one endocrine therapy might be used. Other treatments might be added to endocrine therapy.

There is one type of surgical endocrine therapy:

> **Bilateral oophorectomy** is surgery to remove both ovaries.

Other main types of endocrine therapy include:

> **Ovarian ablation** uses radiation to permanently stop the ovaries from making hormones.

> **Ovarian suppression** uses drugs to temporarily stop the ovaries from making hormones. It is achieved with drugs called LHRH agonists. These drugs stop LHRH from being made, which stops the ovaries from making hormones. LHRH agonists include goserelin (Zoladex) and leuprolide (Lupron Depot). Gonadotropin-releasing hormone (GnRH) agonists might be used to suppress ovarian hormone or testosterone production.

> **Aromatase inhibitors (AIs)** stop a type of hormone called androgen from changing into estrogen by interfering with an enzyme called aromatase. They do not affect estrogen made by the ovaries. Non-steroidal aromatase inhibitors include anastrozole (Arimidex) and letrozole (Femara). Exemestane (Aromasin) is a steroidal aromatase inhibitor.

> **Estrogen receptor (ER) modulators or anti-estrogens** prevent hormones from binding to receptors.

  · **Selective estrogen receptor modulators (SERMs)** block estrogen from attaching to hormone receptors. They include tamoxifen and toremifene (Fareston).

  · **Selective estrogen receptor degraders (SERDs)** block and destroy estrogen receptors. Fulvestrant (Faslodex) is a SERD.

> **Gonadotropin-releasing hormone (GnRH) agonists** might be used to suppress ovarian hormone or testosterone production.

> **Hormones** may be used to treat breast cancer when taken in high doses. It is not known how hormones stop breast cancer from growing. They include ethinyl estradiol, fluoxymesterone, and megestrol acetate (Megace ES).

Those who want to have children in the future should be referred to a fertility specialist to discuss the options before starting chemotherapy and/or endocrine therapy.

Menopausal status

Options for endocrine therapy are partly based on if you started or were in menopause before beginning treatment. In menopause, the ovaries permanently stop producing hormones and menstrual periods stop. After menopause, estrogen and progesterone levels continue to stay low.

Premenopause

If you have menstrual periods, you are in premenopause. In premenopause, the ovaries are the main source of estrogen and progesterone. Tamoxifen is the endocrine treatment for those in premenopause.

Menopause

Cancer treatment can cause a temporary menopause. When menstrual periods stop for 12 months or more, it is called menopause. If you don't have periods, a test using a blood sample may be needed to confirm your status. Menstrual periods may stop during treatment and for up to 2 years after treatment, but often returns in those 40 years of age and under. In menopause, your adrenal glands, liver, and body fat make small amounts of estrogen.

Tamoxifen or an aromatase inhibitor is the endocrine treatment for those in menopause. Aromatase inhibitors include anastrozole (Arimidex), exemestane (Aromasin) and letrozole (Femara).

Testosterone

For those assigned male at birth whose bodies continue to make testosterone, endocrine therapy includes tamoxifen or an aromatase inhibitor with testosterone-suppressing therapy.

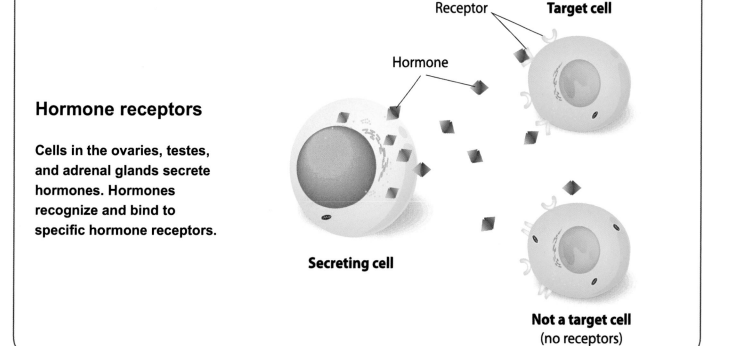

Hormone receptors

Cells in the ovaries, testes, and adrenal glands secrete hormones. Hormones recognize and bind to specific hormone receptors.

Bone-strengthening therapy

Medicines that target the bones may be given to help relieve bone pain or reduce the risk of bone problems. Some medicines work by slowing or stopping bone breakdown, while others help increase bone thickness.

When breast cancer spreads to distant sites, it may metastasize in your bones. This puts your bones at risk for injury and disease. Such problems include bone loss (osteoporosis), fractures, bone pain, and squeezing (compression) of the spinal cord. Some treatments for breast cancer, like endocrine therapy, can cause bone loss, which put you at an increased risk for fractures.

Drugs used to prevent bone loss and fractures:

> ➤ Oral bisphosphonates

> ➤ Zoledronic acid (Zometa)

> ➤ Pamidronate (Aredia)

> ➤ Denosumab (Prolia)

Drugs used to treat bone metastases:

> ➤ Zoledronic acid (Zometa)

> ➤ Pamidronate (Aredia)

> ➤ Denosumab (Xgeva)

You will be screened for bone weakness (osteoporosis) using a bone mineral density test. This measures how much calcium and other minerals are in your bones. It is also called a dual-energy x-ray absorptiometry (DEXA) scan and is painless. Bone mineral density tests look for osteoporosis and help predict your risk for bone fractures.

A baseline DEXA scan is recommended before starting endocrine therapy.

Zoledronic acid, pamidronate, and denosumab

Zoledronic acid, pamidronate, and denosumab are used to prevent bone loss (osteoporosis) and fractures caused by endocrine therapy. Zoledronic acid and denosumab and are also used in those with metastatic breast cancer who have bone metastases to help prevent fractures or spinal cord compression. You might have blood tests to monitor kidney function, calcium levels, and magnesium levels. A calcium and vitamin D supplement will be recommended by your doctor.

Let your dentist know if you are taking any of these medicines. Also, ask your doctor how these medicines might affect your teeth and jaw. Osteonecrosis, or bone tissue death of the jaw, is a rare but serious side effect. Tell your doctor about any planned trips to the dentist and surgeries or dental procedures that might also affect the jaw bone. It will be important to take care of your teeth and to see a dentist before starting treatment with any of these drugs.

Inhibitors

CDK4/6 inhibitors

Cyclin-dependent kinase (CDK) is a cell protein that helps cells grow and divide. For hormone receptor-positive (HR+), HER2- cancer, taking a CDK4/6 inhibitor with endocrine therapy may help control cancer longer. With all CDK4/6 regimens, those who are premenopausal must also receive ovarian ablation or suppression. CDK4/6 inhibitors include abemaciclib (Verzenio), palbociclib (Ibrance), and ribociclib (Kisqali).

A Ki-67 test might be done before adjuvant abemaciclib. Ki-67 is a protein in cells that increases as they prepare to divide into new cells.

EGFR inhibitors

An EGRF inhibitor blocks the activity of a protein called epidermal growth factor receptor (EGFR). Lapatinib (Tykerb) and Neratinib (Nerlynx) are examples of an EGFR inhibitor.

mTOR inhibitors

mTOR is a cell protein that helps cells grow and divide. Endocrine therapy may stop working if mTOR becomes overactive. mTOR inhibitors are used to get endocrine therapy working again.

Everolimus (Afinitor) is an mTOR inhibitor. Most often, it is taken with exemestane. For some, it may be taken with fulvestrant or tamoxifen.

PARP inhibitors

Cancer cells often become damaged. PARP is a cell protein that repairs cancer cells and allows them to survive. Blocking PARP can cause cancer cells to die. Olaparib (Lynparza) and talazoparib (Talzenna) are PARP inhibitors. You must have the *BRCA1* or *BRCA2* mutation and your breast cancer must be HER2- for PARP inhibitors to be effective.

PIK3CA inhibitor

The *PIK3CA* gene is one of the most frequently mutated genes in breast cancers. A mutation in this gene can lead to increased growth of cancer cells and resistance to various treatments. Alpelisib (Piqray) is an example of a PIK3CA inhibitor.

Immunotherapy

Immunotherapy is a type of systemic treatment that increases the activity of your immune system. By doing so, it improves your body's ability to find and destroy cancer cells. Immunotherapy can be given alone or with other types of treatment. Pembrolizumab (Keytruda) and dostarlimab-gxly (Jemperli) target MSI-H or dMMR tumors, or those that express PD-1 or PD-L1. Pembrolizumab also targets tumors that are mutational burden-high (TMB-H).

Clinical trials

A clinical trial is a type of medical research study. After being developed and tested in a laboratory, potential new ways of fighting cancer need to be studied in people. If found to be safe and effective in a clinical trial, a drug, device, or treatment approach may be approved by the U.S. Food and Drug Administration (FDA).

Everyone with cancer should carefully consider all of the treatment options available for their cancer type, including standard treatments and clinical trials. Talk to your doctor about whether a clinical trial may make sense for you.

Phases
Most cancer clinical trials focus on treatment. Treatment trials are done in phases.

> **Phase I trials** study the dose, safety, and side effects of an investigational drug or treatment approach. They also look for early signs that the drug or approach is helpful.

> **Phase II trials** study how well the drug or approach works against a specific type of cancer.

> **Phase III trials** test the drug or approach against a standard treatment. If the results are good, it may be approved by the FDA.

> **Phase IV trials** study the long-term safety and benefit of an FDA-approved treatment.

Who can enroll?
Every clinical trial has rules for joining, called eligibility criteria. The rules may be about age, cancer type and stage, treatment history, or general health. These requirements ensure that participants are alike in specific ways and that the trial is as safe as possible for the participants.

Informed consent
Clinical trials are managed by a group of experts called a research team. The research team will review the study with you in detail, including its purpose and the risks and benefits of joining. All of this information is also provided in an informed consent form. Read the form carefully and ask questions before signing it. Take time to discuss with family, friends, or others whom you trust. Keep in mind that you can leave and seek treatment outside of the clinical trial at any time.

Start the conversation
Don't wait for your doctor to bring up clinical trials. Start the conversation and learn about all of your treatment options. If you find a study that you may be eligible for, ask your treatment team if you meet the requirements. If you have already started standard treatment you may not be eligible for certain clinical trials. Try not to be discouraged if you cannot join. New clinical trials are always becoming available.

Frequently asked questions

There are many myths and misconceptions surrounding clinical trials. The possible benefits and risks are not well understood by many with cancer.

Will I get a placebo?

Placebos (inactive versions of real medicines) are almost never used alone in cancer clinical trials. It is common to receive either a placebo with a standard treatment, or a new drug with a standard treatment. You will be informed, verbally and in writing, if a placebo is part of a clinical trial before you enroll.

Are clinical trials free?

There is no fee to enroll in a clinical trial. The study sponsor pays for research-related costs, including the study drug. You may, however, have costs indirectly related to the trial, such as the cost of transportation or child care due to extra appointments. During the trial, you will continue to receive standard cancer care. This care is billed to—and often covered by—insurance. You are responsible for copays and any costs for this care that are not covered by your insurance.

Finding a clinical trial

In the United States
NCCN Cancer Centers
NCCN.org/cancercenters

The National Cancer Institute (NCI)
cancer.gov/about-cancer/treatment/clinical-trials/search

Worldwide

The U.S. National Library of Medicine (NLM)
clinicaltrials.gov

Need help finding a clinical trial?
NCI's Cancer Information Service (CIS)
1.800.4.CANCER (1.800.422.6237)
cancer.gov/contact

Supportive care

Supportive care is health care given during all cancer stages. It aims to prevent, reduce, and relieve suffering, and to improve quality of life. Supportive care might include pain relief (palliative care), emotional or spiritual support, financial aid, or family counseling. Tell your care team how you are feeling and about any side effects so they can be managed. Best supportive care, supportive care, and palliative care are often used interchangeably.

It is very important to take care of yourself by eating well, drinking plenty of fluids, exercising, and doing things that make you feel energized. Strength is needed to sustain you during treatment.

Bone health

Breast cancer may spread to your bones. Some breast cancer treatments may also weaken your bones. Both of these can put your bones at increased risk for injury and disease. Such problems include bone fractures, bone pain, and squeezing (compression) of the spinal cord. High levels of calcium in the blood, called hypercalcemia, may also occur.

Medicine may be given to help relieve bone pain and reduce the risk of other bone problems. Some medicines work by slowing or stopping bone breakdown, while others help increase bone thickness. It is recommended that you take calcium and vitamin D with these bone health medicines. Talk to your doctor first.

Breastfeeding

Breastfeeding following a lumpectomy is possible. The quantity and quality of breastmilk produced by the breast may not be sufficient or may be lacking some of the nutrients needed. Breastfeeding is not recommended during active treatment or within 6 months of completing certain types of endocrine therapy.

Distress

Distress is an unpleasant experience of a mental, physical, social, or spiritual nature. It can affect how you feel, think, and act. Distress might include feelings of sadness, fear, helplessness, worry, anger, and guilt.

Depression, anxiety, and sleeping problems are common in cancer. Talk to your doctor and with those whom you feel most comfortable about how you are feeling. There are services and people who can help you. Support and counseling services are available.

For more information, see *NCCN Guidelines for Patients: Distress During Cancer Care*, available at NCCN.org/patientguidelines.

Fatigue

Fatigue is extreme tiredness and inability to function due to lack of energy. Fatigue may be caused by cancer or it may be a side effect of treatment. Let your care team know how you are feeling and if fatigue is getting in the way of doing the things you enjoy. Eating a balanced diet, exercise, yoga, and massage therapy can help. You might be referred to a nutritionist or dietitian to help with fatigue.

Hair loss

Chemotherapy may cause hair loss (alopecia) all over your body — not just on your scalp. Some chemotherapy drugs are more likely than others to cause hair loss. Dosage might also affect the amount of hair loss. Most of the time, hair loss from chemotherapy is temporary. Hair often regrows 3 to 6 months after treatment ends. Your hair may be a different shade or texture.

Scalp cooling

Scalp cooling (or scalp hypothermia) might help lessen hair loss in those receiving certain types of chemotherapy. Some people find scalp cooling uncomfortable and have headaches as a side effect from the cold. You may experience hair loss even with scalp cooling treatment.

Low blood cell counts

Some cancer treatments can cause low blood cell counts.

> **Anemia** is a condition where your body does not make enough healthy blood cells, resulting in less oxygen being carried to your cells.

> **Neutropenia** is a decrease in neutrophils, the most common type of white blood cell. This puts you at risk for infection.

> **Thrombocytopenia** is a condition where there are not enough platelets found in the blood.

For more information on anemia, neutropenia, and thrombocytopenia, see *NCCN Guidelines for Patients: Anemia and Neutropenia*, available at NCCN.org/patientguidelines.

Lymphedema

Lymphedema is a condition in which extra lymph fluid builds up in tissues and causes swelling. It may be caused when part of the lymph system is damaged or blocked, such as during surgery to remove lymph nodes, or radiation therapy. Cancers that block lymph vessels can also cause lymphedema. Swelling usually develops slowly over time. It may develop during treatment or it may start years after treatment. If you have lymphedema, you may be referred to an expert in lymphedema management. The swelling may be reduced by exercise, massage, compression sleeves, and other means. Ask your care team about the ways to treat lymphedema.

Nausea and vomiting

Nausea and vomiting are a common side effect of treatment. You will be given medicine to prevent and treat nausea and vomiting.

For more information, see *NCCN Guidelines for Patients: Nausea and Vomiting*, available at NCCN.org/patientguidelines.

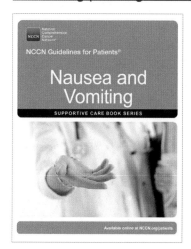

Pain

Tell your care team about any pain or discomfort. You might meet with a palliative care specialist or with a pain specialist to manage pain.

Treatment side effects

All cancer treatments can cause unwanted health issues. Such health issues are called side effects. Side effects depend on many factors. These factors include the drug type and dose, length of treatment, and the person. Some side effects may be harmful to your health. Others may just be unpleasant.

Ask for a complete list of side effects of your treatments. Also, tell your treatment team about any new or worsening symptoms. There may be ways to help you feel better. There are also ways to prevent some side effects.

Trouble eating

Sometimes side effects from surgery, cancer, or other treatments might cause you to feel not hungry or sick to your stomach (nauseated). You might have a sore mouth. Healthy eating is important during treatment. It includes eating a balanced diet, eating the right amount of food, and drinking enough fluids. A registered dietitian who is an expert in nutrition and food can help. Speak to your care team if you have trouble eating or maintaining your weight.

Keep a pain diary

A pain diary is a written record that helps you keep track of when you have pain, how bad it is, what causes it, and what makes it better or worse. Use a pain diary to discuss your pain with your care team. You might be referred to a specialist for pain management.

Include in your pain diary:

- The time and dose of all medicines

- When pain starts and ends or lessens

- Where you feel pain

- Describe your pain. Is it throbbing, sharp, tingling, shooting, or burning? Is it constant, or does it come and go?

- Does the pain change at different times of day? When?

- Does the pain get worse before or after meals? Does certain food or drink make it better?

- Does the pain get better or worse with activity? What kind of activity?

- Does the pain keep you from falling asleep at night? Does pain wake you up in the night?

- Rate your pain from 0 (no pain) to 10 (worst pain you have ever felt)

- Does pain get in the way of you doing the things you enjoy?

Key points

- Treatment takes a team approach. Get to know your care team and let them get to know you.

- Invasive breast cancer is treatable. The goal of treatment is to remove the tumor, when possible, and prevent or slow the spread of cancer.

- Treatment for invasive breast cancer is a combination of therapies.

- Local therapy focuses on a certain area. It includes surgery, ablation, and radiation therapy.

- Systemic therapy works throughout the body. It includes endocrine therapy, chemotherapy, and targeted therapy.

- A sentinel lymph node (SLN) is the first lymph node that cancer cells are most likely to spread to from a primary tumor. A sentinel lymph node biopsy (SNLB) might be done to look for cancer.

- A lumpectomy is also called breast-conserving surgery (BCS).

- A total mastectomy or a simple mastectomy is a surgery that removes the whole breast.

- A skin-sparing mastectomy removes the breast but not all the skin.

- A nipple-sparing mastectomy preserves the nipple areola complex (NAC). Not everyone is a candidate for nipple-sparing mastectomy.

- Those who want to have children in the future should be referred to a fertility specialist before starting chemotherapy and/or endocrine therapy to discuss the options.

> It is important to tell your care team about all side effects so they can be managed.

- A clinical trial is a type of research that studies a treatment to see how safe it is and how well it works.

- Supportive care is health care that relieves symptoms caused by cancer or its treatment and improves quality of life. Supportive care is always given.

- All cancer treatments can cause unwanted health issues called side effects. It is important for you to tell your care team about all your side effects so they can be managed.

- Eating a balanced diet, drinking enough fluids, exercise, yoga, and massage therapy can help manage side effects.

5
The breast after surgery

53 Volume displacement

53 Flat closure

53 Breast reconstruction

54 Nipple replacement

55 What to consider

56 Key points

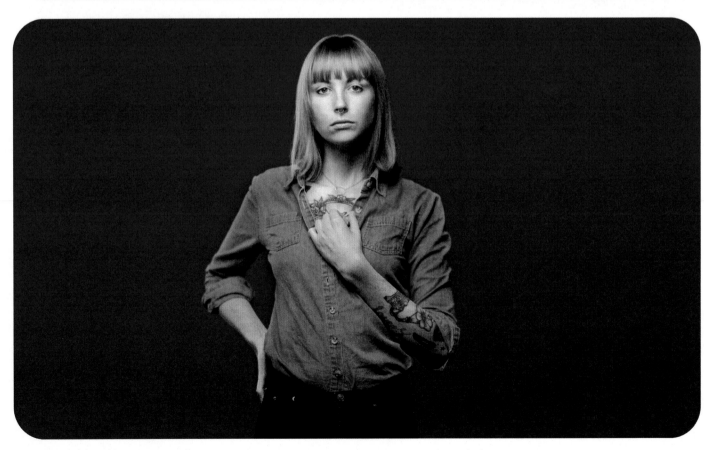

The look of your breast after surgery will depend on the type of surgery, the amount of tissue removed, and other factors such as your body type, age, and size and shape of the area before surgery. This chapter offers more information on volume displacement, flat closure, and breast reconstruction.

Volume displacement

With a lumpectomy, most people have a scar with some volume loss, but are satisfied with the way their breast looks. However, if you need a large lumpectomy and your surgeon thinks your breast will look more abnormal afterwards, your breast may be able to be re-shaped at the time of surgery. This procedure is called volume displacement or oncoplasty. It is often done by the cancer surgeon or plastic surgeon right after the lumpectomy. The surgeon will shift the remaining breast tissue to fill the gap left by the removed tumor.

If volume displacement is planned, a larger piece of your breast will need to be removed. Despite a larger piece being removed, the natural look of your breast will be kept.

You may not like the results of the volume displacement. In this case, breast revision surgery may help. This surgery is done by a plastic surgeon. A second volume displacement may be an option, too. Another option is to get breast implants or mastectomy with reconstruction.

Flat closure

In a total mastectomy with a flat closure, the entire breast, including nipple, extra skin, fat, and other tissue in the breast area are removed. The remaining skin is tightened and sewn together. No breast mound is created and no implant is added. The scar will be slightly raised and differ in color than the surrounding skin. A flat closure is not completely flat or smooth. The end result varies from person to person depending on their body and fat tissue. Ask to look at "after" pictures from flat closures so you know what to expect.

You might decide to have a flat closure procedure at a later time or after having breast implants removed. Talk to your care team to learn more.

Breast reconstruction

Breast reconstruction is surgery to rebuild the shape and look of the breast after a mastectomy. In many cases, breast reconstruction involves a staged approach. It might require more than one procedure.

You may have a choice as to when breast reconstruction is done. Immediate reconstruction is finished within hours after removing the breast. Delayed reconstruction can occur months or years after the cancer surgery. Reconstruction can also be done in a staged fashion, with part of the reconstruction done at the time of the original cancer surgery, and finished with another surgery at a later time. A plastic surgeon performs breast reconstruction.

Breasts can be reconstructed with implants and flaps. All methods are generally safe, but as with any surgery, there are risks. Ask your treatment team for a complete list of side effects.

Implants

Breast implants are small bags filled with salt water, silicone gel, or both. They are placed under the breast skin or muscle to look like a new breast. A balloon-like device, called an expander, may be used first to stretch out tissue. It will be placed under your skin or muscle and enlarged every few weeks for two to three months. When your skin is stretched to the proper size, you will have surgery to place the final implant.

Implants have a small risk of leaking or causing other issues. You may feel pain from the implant or expander. Scar tissue or tissue death can occur. Textured implants can cause breast implant-associated anaplastic large cell lymphoma (BIA-ALCL), a type of cancer.

Flaps

Sometimes breast fullness can be recreated after a skin-sparing mastectomy. In a skin-sparing mastectomy, breast tissue is removed from underneath the skin. The nipple remains intact, if possible. The remaining skin flaps are used to create a breast mound. This technique does not use implants or skin transferred from other parts of the body and may be completed in a single surgery. This is best suited for those with larger breasts who are willing to have much smaller breasts as a result.

Breasts can be remade using tissue from other parts of your body, known as "flaps." These flaps are taken from the belly, butt, thigh, or from under the shoulder blade. Some flaps are completely removed and then sewn in place. Other flaps stay attached to your body but are slid over and sewn into place.

Flaps can cause problems. There may be tissue death which can cause lumps. A hernia may occur from muscle weakness. Problems are more likely to occur among those who have diabetes or who smoke.

Implants and flaps

Some breasts are reconstructed with both implants and flaps. This method may give the reconstructed breast more volume to match the other breast. For any reconstruction, you may need surgery on your remaining breast to match the two breasts in size and shape.

Nipple replacement

Like your breast, a nipple can be remade. To rebuild a nipple, a plastic surgeon can use surrounding tissues. Also, nipples can be remade with tissue from the thigh, other nipple, or the sex organs between your legs (vulva). Tissue can be darkened with a tattoo to look more like a nipple. It is important to note that while you can remake something to look like a nipple, it will not have the sensation of your real nipple. Also, a tattoo can be done to look like a nipple without having to take tissue from another part of the body.

What to consider

Some things to consider when deciding to have flat closure or reconstruction after mastectomy:

> **Your desire** – You may have a strong feeling towards flat closure or one form of reconstruction after being given the options. Breast reconstruction should be a shared decision between you and your care team. Make your wishes known.

> **Health issues** – You may have health issues such as diabetes or a blood disorder that might affect or delay healing, or make longer procedures unsafe.

> **Tobacco use** – Smoking delays wound healing and can cause mastectomy flap death (necrosis), nipple-areola complex (NAC) necrosis in a nipple-sparing mastectomy, infection, and failure of implant-based reconstruction. In free flap reconstruction, smoking increases the risk of complications. Ask for help if you smoke and might consider trying to quit. You are encouraged to stop smoking prior to reconstruction.

> **Breast size and shape** – There are limits to the available sizes of breast implants. Very large breasts or breasts that lack tone or droop (called ptosis) might be difficult to match. Breast reduction surgery might be an option.

> **Body mass index (BMI)** – Those with an elevated BMI have increased risk of infections and complications with breast reconstruction.

Tattoo

Removed nipples can be remade with body tissue and/or tattooing.

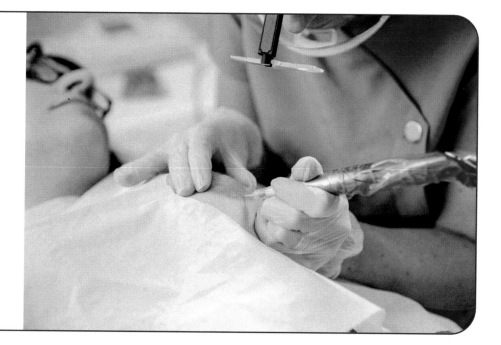

Key points

- Volume displacement is a shifting of the breast tissue to fill the gap left by a lumpectomy.

- Flat closure is done after a mastectomy in which the skin is tightened and sewn together without the addition of a breast implant.

- Breast reconstruction is surgery to rebuild the shape and look of the breast.

- Breasts that are fully removed in a mastectomy can be remade with breast implants, flaps, or both.

- Removed nipples can be remade with body tissue and/or tattooing.

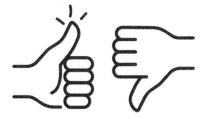

Let us know what you think!

Please take a moment to complete an online survey about the NCCN Guidelines for Patients.

NCCN.org/patients/response

6
Stages 1, 2, and 3A

58	Surgery and radiation therapy
59	Adjuvant systemic therapy
60	HR+ with HER2+
61	HR+ with HER2-
62	HR- with HER2+
63	HR- with HER2-
64	Adjuvant endocrine therapy
65	Follow-up care
66	Key points

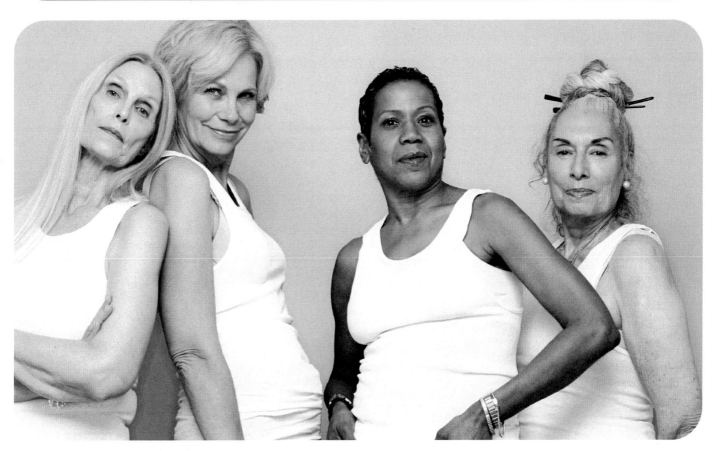

Surgery is the main or primary treatment for invasive breast cancer. Treatment before surgery is called preoperative therapy. Not all cancers need treatment before surgery. This chapter is for those who will not have preoperative therapy. Together, you and your doctor will choose the best option for you.

Not all cancers need treatment before surgery. If your doctor is considering treatment before surgery (preoperative), then Chapter 7 is where you can find that information. This chapter is for those who will not have preoperative therapy.

Surgery and radiation therapy

Surgery is the main or primary treatment for invasive breast cancer. It involves removing the tumor from the breast and assessing the lymph nodes.

There are 2 breast surgery options:

> Lumpectomy

> Total mastectomy

Both options include axillary lymph node (ALN) staging with either sentinel lymph node biopsy (SLNB) or axillary lymph node dissection (ALND) or both. After surgery, a pathologist will examine the removed tissue and any lymph nodes to determine the pathologic stage. This information will help plan next steps for treatment. Treatment after surgery might include radiation therapy and/or systemic therapy.

An example of a tumor stage after surgery might be pT2. Lymph node micrometastases are written as pN1mi. Ipsilateral means on the same side of the body.

Lumpectomy

A lumpectomy, also called breast-conserving surgery (BCS), is surgery to remove a tumor in the breast. Treatment after a lumpectomy is based on the type of cancer and if cancer is found in the axillary lymph nodes (ALNs). If there is a positive surgical margin, you might have more surgery to remove any remaining cancer. Whole breast radiation therapy (WBRT) is usually recommended after a lumpectomy. Regional node irradiation (RNI) might be added. Chemotherapy might be given before RT.

Total mastectomy

A total mastectomy is a surgery that removes the whole breast. Treatment after a mastectomy is based on if cancer was found in the axillary lymph nodes (ALNs), the number of lymph nodes that tested positive, and the size of the removed tumor. Radiation therapy and/or systemic therapy are possible following a mastectomy.

Adjuvant systemic therapy

Drug treatment after surgery or radiation therapy is called adjuvant systemic therapy. It is given to kill any remaining cancer cells and to help reduce the risk of cancer returning. This treatment is based on cancer subtype called tumor histology and hormone receptor (HR) status. Histology is the study of the anatomy (structure) of cells, tissues, and organs under a microscope. Depending on the histology, HER2 status may also be a factor. If cancer is hormone receptor-positive (ER+ and/or PR+) and HER2-, then oncologists also take into account if there is cancer in lymph nodes called node positive (node+).

Systemic therapies might be used alone or in combination. Ask your medical oncologist why one treatment might be preferred over another for your type of cancer.

For those in menopause (natural or induced) with high-risk node-negative or node-positive tumors, bone-strengthening therapy might be given to reduce the risk of distant metastasis.

Favorable histologies

A favorable histology is one that has a favorable or good prognosis. A prognosis is the course your cancer will likely take. These tumor types are not high grade, are HER2-, and might respond better to treatment than other tumors. They also might have less risk of returning. Ask your doctor what this might mean for your treatment. Those with estrogen receptor-positive (ER+) and/or progesterone receptor-positive (PR+) tumors will likely have endocrine therapy. Other systemic therapies are possible.

Favorable histology types include:

> Pure tubular

> Pure mucinous

> Pure cribriform

> Encapsulated or solid papillary carcinoma

> Adenoid cystic and other salivary carcinomas

> Secretory carcinoma

> Rare low-grade forms of metaplastic carcinoma

> Other rare forms

Common histologies

Ductal and lobular carcinoma are the most common types of invasive breast cancer.

Common histology types include:

> Ductal/NST (NST includes medullary pattern, cancers with neuroendocrine expression, and other rare patterns)

> Lobular

> Mixed

> Micropapillary

> Metaplastic

Adjuvant treatment options for common histologies are described next.

HR+ with HER2+

In hormone receptor-positive (HR+) cancer, estrogen (ER+) and/or progesterone receptors (PR+) are found. If HER2 receptors are found, the cancer is also HER2+. It might be written as HR+ with HER2+ or called triple-positive breast cancer.

Endocrine therapy is used to treat HR+ breast cancer. Chemotherapy with a HER2-targeted therapy is used to treat HER2+ cancer. Examples of HER2-targeted therapy used after surgery include trastuzumab and pertuzumab.

Systemic therapies might be used alone or in combination. If chemotherapy is given, it is given before endocrine therapy. Ask your medical oncologist why one treatment might be preferred over another for your type of cancer.

Adjuvant (after surgery) systemic treatment options for HR+ with HER2+ are found in Guide 3.

Guide 3 Adjuvant therapy options: HR+ and HER2+	
Lymph node negative (pN0) or micrometastasis (pN1mi) of 2 mm or less	If tumor is 0.5 cm or less and no cancer in lymph nodes, consider: • Endocrine therapy • Endocrine therapy with chemotherapy and trastuzumab
	If tumor is 0.5 cm or less and micrometastasis: • Endocrine therapy • Chemotherapy with trastuzumab and endocrine therapy
	If tumor is 0.6 cm to 1 cm: • Endocrine therapy • Chemotherapy with trastuzumab and endocrine therapy
	If tumor is larger than 1 cm: • Chemotherapy with trastuzumab and endocrine therapy
Lymph node positive (pN+) for 1 or more metastases larger than 2 mm	Options are: • Chemotherapy with trastuzumab and endocrine therapy • Chemotherapy with trastuzumab, pertuzumab, and endocrine therapy

HR+ with HER2-

In hormone receptor-positive (HR+) cancer, estrogen (ER+) and/or progesterone receptors (PR+) are found. Endocrine therapy is used to treat HR+ breast cancer. Since there are no HER2 receptors, therapy targeting the HER2 receptors is not used. Often, chemotherapy is used instead. When cancer is found in the lymph nodes, it is node positive (node+).

> Those who are premenopausal might have ovarian suppression or ablation in addition to endocrine therapy.

> If chemotherapy is given, it is given before endocrine therapy.

Chemotherapy and other systemic therapies specific to HER2- are found in Guide 4.

Guide 4 **Adjuvant systemic therapy options: HER2-**	
Preferred options	• Doxorubicin and cyclophosphamide followed by paclitaxel • Docetaxel and cyclophosphamide (TC) • Olaparib, if germline *BRCA1* or *BRCA2* mutations
	• High-risk triple-negative breast cancer (TNBC): Preoperative pembrolizumab with carboplatin and paclitaxel, followed by preoperative pembrolizumab andcyclophosphamide with doxorubicin or epirubicin, followed by adjuvant pembrolizumab • If TNBC and residual disease after preoperative therapy with taxane-, alkylator-, and anthracycline-based chemotherapy, then capecitabine
Other recommended	• Doxorubicin and cyclophosphamide followed by docetaxel • Epirubicin and cyclophosphamide (EC) • Docetaxel, doxorubicin, and cyclophosphamide (TAC)
	Only in certain TNBC cases: • Paclitaxel with carboplatin • Docetaxel with carboplatin (preoperative setting only)
Used in some cases	• Doxorubicin and cyclophosphamide • Cyclophosphamide, methotrexate, and fluorouracil (CMF) • Doxorubicin and cyclophosphamide followed by paclitaxel • Capecitabine (maintenance therapy for TNBC after adjuvant chemotherapy)

HR- with HER2+

In hormone receptor-negative (HR-) cancer, there are no receptors for estrogen (ER-) and progesterone (PR-). When HER2 receptors are found, it is HER2-positive (HER2+). Since this cancer is HR- and HER2+, treatment will focus on targeting HER2. HER2-targeted therapy usually includes chemotherapy.

HER2-targeted therapy options can be found in Guide 5.

Did you know?

The terms "chemotherapy" and "systemic therapy" are often used interchangeably, but they are not the same. Chemotherapy, targeted therapy, and immunotherapy are all types of systemic therapy.

Guide 5
Adjuvant HER2-targeted therapy (HER2+) options

Preferred options	• Paclitaxel and trastuzumab • Docetaxel, carboplatin, and trastuzumab (TCH) • Docetaxel, carboplatin, trastuzumab, and pertuzumab (TCHP) • Complete up to 1 year of HER2-targeted therapy with trastuzumab. Pertuzumab might be added.
Other recommended	• Doxorubicin with cyclophosphamide followed by docetaxel with trastuzumab • Doxorubicin with cyclophosphamide followed by docetaxel with trastuzumab and pertuzumab
Used in some cases	• Docetaxel, cyclophosphamide, and trastuzumab • Doxorubicin and cyclophosphamide followed by paciltaxel with trastuzumab • Doxorubicin and cyclophosphamide followed by docetaxel with paclitaxel, trastuzumab, and pertuzumab • Neratinib • Paclitaxel with trastuzumab and pertuzumab • Ado-trastuzumab emtansine (TDM-1)

Note: An FDA-approved biosimilar might be used for trastuzumab.

HR- with HER2-

In triple-negative breast cancer (TNBC), receptors for estrogen, progesterone, and HER2 are not found. This means that the breast cancer cells have tested negative for HER2 and both hormone receptors. It is written as ER- and/or PR- with HER2-.

TNBC is cancer that is:

> Estrogen receptor-negative (ER-),

> Progesterone receptor-negative (PR-), and

> HER2-negative (HER2-).

There are many variations within TNBC. It is a group of diseases that we are learning more about all the time. Since there are no HER2 receptors, HER2- targeted therapy is not used. And since there are no estrogen or progesterone hormone receptors, endocrine therapy is not used. Adjuvant treatment will likely be chemotherapy as found in Guide 4.

Order of treatments

Most people with breast cancer will receive more than one type of treatment. Below is an overview of the order of treatments.

- **Preoperative or neoadjuvant (before) therapy** is given to shrink the tumor before primary treatment (surgery).

- **Perioperative therapy** is systemic therapy, such as chemotherapy, given before and after surgery.

- **Primary treatment** is the main treatment given to rid the body of cancer. Surgery is often the main treatment for invasive breast cancer.

- **Postoperative or adjuvant (after) therapy** is given after primary treatment to rid the body of any cancer cells left behind from surgery. It is also used when the risk of cancer returning (recurrence) is felt to be high.

- **Definitive treatment** is defined as the best treatment after all choices have been considered.

- **First-line therapy** is the first set of systemic (drug) treatment given.

- **Second-line therapy** is the next set of treatment given if cancer progresses during or after systemic therapy.

Talk to your doctor about your treatment plan and what it means for your stage and type of breast cancer.

Adjuvant endocrine therapy

Adjuvant endocrine therapy is used to treat hormone receptor-positive (HR+) breast cancer. This is cancer that tests positive for estrogen receptors (ER+) and/or progesterone receptors (PR+). Endocrine therapy blocks estrogen and progesterone, which can slow tumor growth or shrink the tumor for a period of time. It might also help prevent the risk of cancer returning in the breasts and elsewhere in the body. If chemotherapy is given, it is given before endocrine therapy.

Those with high-risk breast cancer that is HER2- might have 2 years of adjuvant abemaciclib with endocrine therapy.

Those receiving an aromatase inhibitor who are at risk for osteoporosis will likely have bone density tests and bone-strengthening therapy.

Adjuvant endocrine therapy options can be found in Guide 6.

Guide 6
Adjuvant endocrine therapy

Premenopause at diagnosis	• Tamoxifen alone for 5 years • Tamoxifen for 5 years with ovarian suppression or ablation →	• After 5 years, if in menopause, then an aromatase inhibitor for 5 years or consider tamoxifen for another 5 years (for a total of 10 years on tamoxifen) • After 5 years, if still in premenopause, then consider tamoxifen for another 5 years (for a total of 10 years on tamoxifen) or stop endocrine therapy
	• Aromatase inhibitor for 5 years with ovarian suppression or ablation. Then consider aromatase inhibitor for an additional 3 to 5 years	
Menopause at diagnosis	• Aromatase inhibitor for 5 years, then consider aromatase inhibitor for 3 to 5 more years • Aromatase inhibitor for 2 to 3 years, then tamoxifen to complete 5 years total of endocrine therapy • Tamoxifen for 2 to 3 years, then an aromatase inhibitor to complete 5 years of endocrine therapy • Tamoxifen for 2 to 3 years, then up to 5 years of an aromatase inhibitor	
	• Tamoxifen for 4.5 to 6 years, then an aromatase inhibitor for 5 years or consider tamoxifen for another 5 years (for a total of 10 years on tamoxifen)	
	• For those who can't have aromatase inhibitors or who don't want aromatase inhibitors, take tamoxifen for 5 years or consider tamoxifen for up to 10 years	

Follow-up care

After treatment, you will enter follow-up care. During this time, your health will be monitored for side effects of treatment and the return of cancer. This is part of your survivorship care plan. It is important to keep any follow-up doctor visits and imaging test appointments. Seek good routine medical care, including regular doctor visits for preventive care and cancer screening.

Tell your doctor about any symptoms such as headaches, menstrual spotting between periods or new onset of spotting after menopause (if prior tamoxifen), shortness of breath that you notice with walking, or bone pain. Side effects can be managed. Continue to take all medicine such as endocrine therapy exactly as prescribed and do not miss or skip doses.

You should receive a personalized survivorship care plan. It will provide a summary of possible long-term effects of treatment and list follow-up tests. Find out how your primary care provider will coordinate with specialists for your follow-up care.

Follow-up care can be found in Guide 7.

Guide 7
Follow-up care

Medical history and physical exam 1 to 4 times per year as needed for 5 years, then every year

Screen for changes in family history

Genetic testing and referral to genetic counseling, as needed

Monitor for lymphedema and refer for lymphedema management, as needed

Mammogram every 12 months (not needed on reconstructed breast)

Heart tests, as needed

If signs and symptoms of metastases, then blood and imaging tests

If on endocrine therapy, continue to take endocrine therapy. Do not miss or skip doses

Annual gynecology exam for those on tamoxifen

Bone density tests for those on an aromatase inhibitor or who later have ovarian failure

Maintain an ideal weight, be active, eat a healthy diet, exercise, limit alcohol, and quit smoking

---

Key points

- Surgery is the main or primary treatment for invasive breast cancer. Radiation therapy (RT) and/or systemic therapy are possible following surgery.

- Treatment after surgery is called adjuvant treatment. It is based on the pathologic stage. During surgery, your tumor is tested to determine the pathologic stage.

- Adjuvant systemic therapy is given after surgery to kill any remaining cancer cells and to help prevent the return of cancer.

- Adjuvant treatment is based on the stage, histology, and hormone receptor status. Histology is the study of the anatomy (structure) of cells, tissues, and organs under a microscope.

- A favorable histology is one that has a favorable or good prognosis.

- In hormone receptor-positive (HR+) cancer, estrogen (ER+) and/or progesterone receptors (PR+) are found.

- Endocrine therapy is used to treat HR+ cancer.

- If chemotherapy is given, it is given before endocrine therapy.

- In triple-negative breast cancer (TNBC), receptors for estrogen, progesterone, and HER2 are not found. It is treated with chemotherapy.

- It is important to keep follow-up visits and imaging test appointments. Seek good routine medical care, including preventative care and cancer screenings. Continue to take all medicines as prescribed.

> Those who want to have children in the future should be referred to a fertility specialist before starting endocrine therapy.

7
Stage 3

68	Overview
68	Testing
69	Tumor is operable
69	Tumor is inoperable
70	Adjuvant treatment
72	Triple-negative breast cancer
73	Adjuvant endocrine therapy
74	Follow-up care
75	Key points

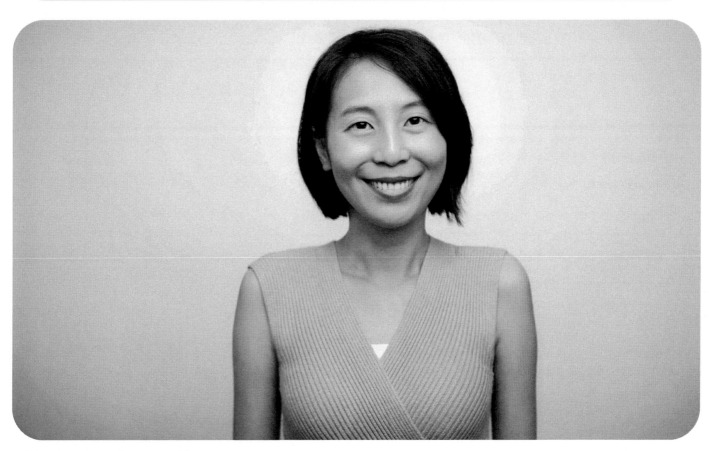

This chapter is for those who have stage 3 breast cancer or for those who would benefit from treatment before surgery. Treatment before surgery is called preoperative or neoadjuvant therapy. It can be systemic therapy or radiation therapy. Preoperative therapy is not for everyone. Together, you and your doctor will choose the best option for you.

Overview

In stage 3 breast cancer, the cancer can be large and in the lymph nodes, the lymph nodes can be fixed (or not moveable), or the cancer can involve the skin or chest wall. It is not metastatic (stage 4).

Treatment before surgery is called preoperative therapy. It can be systemic (drug) therapy or radiation therapy. Preoperative systemic therapy has benefits.

It can:

> Help preserve the breast

> Shrink the tumor

> Shrink the tumor so it can be removed with a smaller surgery (lumpectomy)

> Provide important information about how your tumor responds to therapy, which is very helpful in those with triple-negative (TNBC) and HER2+ breast cancer

> Help choose adjuvant regimens in those with HER2+ and TNBC with residual disease

> Allow time for genetic testing

> Allow time to plan breast reconstruction in those choosing mastectomy

> Allow time for fewer lymph nodes to be removed at the time of surgery

> Allow time for you to decide about and prepare for surgery

There are risks with any treatment. While rare, cancer can still progress during preoperative systemic therapy.

Testing

Not everyone will benefit from preoperative therapy. If preoperative systemic therapy is an option for you, then you will have blood and imaging tests before starting treatment. These tests will determine if your cancer can be removed with surgery (operable) or cannot be removed with surgery at this time (inoperable). Testing will include axillary lymph node exam with ultrasound and biopsy of lymph nodes suspected of cancer.

Tumor is operable

Drug therapy before surgery is called preoperative systemic therapy. This section is for a tumor that can be removed with surgery and will be treated with preoperative therapy.

You will have the following before starting preoperative systemic therapy:

> Core biopsy of breast

> Placement of clips or markers to help the surgeon know where to operate in case the tumor goes away with preoperative therapy. Clips are placed at the time of surgery for radiation planning.

> Axillary lymph node ultrasound or MRI (if not done before)

> Biopsy of suspicious lymph nodes with clip placement

Systemic therapy

Before surgery (preoperative) systemic therapy is based on hormone receptor (HR) and HER2 status. The systemic therapy options are the same as for after surgery (adjuvant) options found on the following pages.

Surgery

Surgery options depend on how your cancer responded to preoperative therapy. A complete response means there is no evidence of cancer. In a partial response, the tumor in the breast or lymph nodes has shrunk in size. A lumpectomy or mastectomy are options depending on the size and location of the tumor. After surgery, most will have both systemic therapy and radiation therapy.

Tumor is inoperable

If initial tests show the tumor cannot be completely removed with surgery (inoperable), then you will have preoperative systemic therapy. Talk with your doctor about what types of preoperative therapy are right for you.

During and after preoperative therapy, you will have tests to monitor treatment. If the tumor shrinks or the cancer burden is reduced, then surgery might be possible.

> If surgery is possible, options are a lumpectomy or mastectomy. Both options include axillary lymph node (ALN) staging. After surgery, a pathologist will examine the removed tissue and any lymph nodes to determine the pathologic stage. Systemic therapy and radiation therapy will follow surgery.

> If the tumor did not shrink enough to be removed with surgery, then you will have more systemic therapy and/or radiation therapy.

Adjuvant treatment

Many people have treatment after surgery. Treatment after surgery is called adjuvant therapy. Adjuvant therapy is based on the size of the tumor, if cancer remains (residual disease), and if cancer in the lymph nodes is found. A complete response means there is no evidence of cancer.

Your tumor will be restaged after preoperative therapy. Staging will be done by looking at tissue removed during surgery. This is called the pathologic stage or surgical stage. It might look like this: ypT0N0. The "y" means you had preoperative therapy.

ER+ and/or PR+ is called hormone receptor-positive (HR+). It is often treated with adjuvant endocrine therapy. HER2-targeted therapy is often used to treat HER2+ cancer. Systemic therapies might be used alone or in combination. When chemotherapy is used, it is given before endocrine therapy. Ask your medical oncologist why one treatment might be preferred over another for your type of cancer.

For those in menopause (natural or induced) with high-risk node-negative or node-positive tumors, bone-strengthening therapy might be given to reduce the risk of distant metastasis.

Guide 9 Adjuvant HER2-targeted therapy (HER2+) options	
Preferred options	• Paclitaxel and trastuzumab • Docetaxel, carboplatin, and trastuzumab (TCH) • Docetaxel, carboplatin, trastuzumab, and pertuzumab (TCHP) • Complete up to one year of HER2-targeted therapy with trastuzumab. Pertuzumab might be added
Other recommended	• Doxorubicin with cyclophosphamide followed by docetaxel with trastuzumab • Doxorubicin with cyclophosphamide followed by docetaxel with trastuzumab and pertuzumab
Used in some cases	• Docetaxel, cyclophosphamide, and trastuzumab • Doxorubicin and cyclophosphamide followed by paciltaxel with trastuzumab • Doxorubicin and cyclophosphamide followed by docetaxel with paclitaxel, trastuzumab, and pertuzumab • Neratinib • Paclitaxel with trastuzumab and pertuzumab • Ado-trastuzumab emtansine (TDM-1)

Note: An FDA-approved biosimilar might be used for trastuzumab.

HR+ with HER2-

ER+ and/or PR+ is called hormone receptor-positive (HR+). It is treated with adjuvant endocrine therapy. Olaparib might be added in some cases.

HR- with HER2+

ER- and/or PR- is called hormone receptor-negative (HR-). Since this cancer is HER2+, it is treated with targeted therapy.

HER2-targeted therapy options can be found in Guide 9.

> ➤ If no disease remains after preoperative therapy, then you will have up to 1 year of HER2-targeted therapy with trastuzumab alone or with pertuzumab.

> ➤ If disease remains in the breast or there is cancer in the lymph nodes (node positive), then you will have ado-trastuzumab emtansine. If ado-trastuzumab emtansine is discontinued for toxicity, then you will receive trastuzumab alone or with pertuzumab to complete 1 year of therapy.

HR+ with HER2+

Hormone receptor-positive (HR+) with HER2+ is also called triple-positive breast cancer. Receptors for HER2, estrogen, and/or progesterone are found. It is treated with HER2-targeted therapy and endocrine therapy.

HER2-targeted therapy options can be found in Guide 9.

> ➤ If no disease remains after preoperative therapy, then you will have endocrine therapy and up to 1 year of HER2-targeted therapy with trastuzumab alone or with pertuzumab.

> ➤ If disease remains or there is cancer in the lymph nodes (node positive), then you will have ado-trastuzumab emtansine. If ado-trastuzumab emtansine was discontinued for toxicity, then trastuzumab alone or with pertuzumab will be given to complete 1 year of therapy. Endocrine therapy will be added.

Triple-negative breast cancer

In triple-negative breast cancer (TNBC), the tumor has tested negative for HER2, estrogen receptors, and progesterone receptors. It is written as ER- and/or PR- with HER2-. This cancer does not respond to endocrine therapy or HER2-targeted therapy. It is treated with chemotherapy and other systemic therapies found in Guide 10.

> If no disease remains after preoperative therapy and are at high risk for the return of cancer, then you will have pembrolizumab (if pembrolizumab-containing regimen was given before surgery).

> If disease remains or there is cancer in the lymph nodes (node positive), then you will have capecitabine. Olaparib might be given if *BRCA1* or *BRCA2* mutation found. Pembrolizumab is an option if pembrolizumab-containing regimen was given before surgery.

Guide 10 Adjuvant systemic therapy options: HER2-	
Preferred options	• Doxorubicin and cyclophosphamide followed by paclitaxel • Docetaxel and cyclophosphamide (TC) • Olaparib, if germline *BRCA1* or *BRCA2* mutations
	• High-risk triple-negative breast cancer (TNBC): Preoperative pembrolizumab with carboplatin and paclitaxel, followed by preoperative pembrolizumab andcyclophosphamide with doxorubicin or epirubicin, followed by adjuvant pembrolizumab • If TNBC and residual disease after preoperative therapy with taxane-, alkylator-, and anthracycline-based chemotherapy, then capecitabine
Other recommended	• Doxorubicin and cyclophosphamide followed by docetaxel • Epirubicin and cyclophosphamide (EC) • Docetaxel, doxorubicin, and cyclophosphamide (TAC)
	Only in certain TNBC cases: • Paclitaxel with carboplatin • Docetaxel with carboplatin (preoperative setting only)
Used in some cases	• Doxorubicin and cyclophosphamide • Cyclophosphamide, methotrexate, and fluorouracil (CMF) • Doxorubicin and cyclophosphamide followed by paclitaxel • Capecitabine (maintenance therapy for TNBC after adjuvant chemotherapy)

Adjuvant endocrine therapy

Adjuvant endocrine therapy is used to treat hormone receptor-positive (HR+) breast cancer. This is cancer that tests positive for estrogen receptors (ER+) and/or progesterone receptors (PR+). Endocrine therapy blocks estrogen and progesterone to treat HR+ breast cancer. This can slow tumor growth or shrink the tumor for a period of time. It might also help prevent the risk of cancer returning.

Endocrine therapy is often used with other systemic therapies.

Adjuvant endocrine therapy options can be found in Guide 11.

Guide 11 Adjuvant endocrine therapy		
Premenopause at diagnosis	• Tamoxifen alone for 5 years • Tamoxifen for 5 years with ovarian suppression or ablation	• After 5 years, if in postmenopause, then an aromatase inhibitor for 5 years or consider tamoxifen for another 5 years (for a total of 10 years on tamoxifen)
		• After 5 years, if still in premenopause, then consider tamoxifen for another 5 years (for a total of 10 years on tamoxifen) or stop endocrine therapy
	• Aromatase inhibitor for 5 years with ovarian suppression or ablation, then consider aromatase inhibitor for an additional 3 to 5 years	
Menopause at diagnosis	• Aromatase inhibitor for 5 years, then consider aromatase inhibitor for 3 to 5 more years • Aromatase inhibitor for 2 to 3 years, then tamoxifen to complete 5 years total of endocrine therapy • Tamoxifen for 2 to 3 years, then an aromatase inhibitor to complete 5 years of endocrine therapy • Tamoxifen for 2 to 3 years, then up to 5 years of an aromatase inhibitor	
	• Tamoxifen for 4.5 to 6 years, then an aromatase inhibitor for 5 years or consider tamoxifen for another 5 years (for a total of 10 years on tamoxifen)	
	• For those who can't have aromatase inhibitors or who don't want aromatase inhibitors, take tamoxifen for 5 years or consider tamoxifen for up to 10 years	

Follow-up care

After treatment, you will enter follow-up care. During this time, your health will be monitored for side effects of treatment and the return of cancer. This is part of your survivorship care plan. It is important to keep any follow-up doctor visits and imaging test appointments and seek good routine medical care, including regular doctor visits for preventive care and cancer screening.

Tell your doctor about any symptoms such as headaches or bone pain. Side effects can be managed. Continue to take all medicine such as endocrine therapy exactly as prescribed and do not miss or skip doses.

You should receive a personalized survivorship care plan. It will provide a summary of possible long-term effects of treatment and list follow-up tests. Find out how your primary care provider will coordinate with specialists for your follow-up care.

Follow-up care can be found in Guide 12.

Guide 12
Follow-up care

Medical history and physical exam 1 to 4 times per year as needed for 5 years, then every year

Screen for changes in family history

Genetic testing and referral to genetic counseling, as needed

Monitor for lymphedema and refer for lymphedema management, as needed

Mammogram every 12 months (not needed on reconstructed breast)

Heart tests, as needed

If signs and symptoms of metastases, then blood and imaging tests

If on endocrine therapy, continue to take endocrine therapy. Do not miss or skip doses.

Annual gynecology exam for those on tamoxifen

Bone density tests for those on an aromatase inhibitor or who later have ovarian failure

Maintain an ideal weight, be active, eat a healthy diet, exercise, limit alcohol, and quit smoking

Key points

- In stage 3 breast cancer, the cancer can be large and in the lymph nodes, the lymph nodes can be fixed (or not moveable), or the cancer can involve the skin or chest wall. It is not metastatic.

- Treatment before surgery is called preoperative therapy. It can be systemic therapy or radiation therapy. The goal of treatment is to shrink the tumor before surgery.

- Systemic therapy after surgery is called adjuvant therapy. Adjuvant therapy is based on how the tumor responded to preoperative treatment.

- All treatment is based on if the tumor has receptors for HER2, estrogen, and/or progesterone.

- In hormone receptor-positive (HR+) breast cancer, tests find hormone receptors for estrogen and/or progesterone on the tumor.

- HR+ breast cancer is treated with endocrine therapy.

- HER2-positive (HER2+) breast cancer is treated with HER2-targeted therapy.

- It is important to keep follow-up visits and imaging test appointments. Seek good routine medical care, including preventative care and cancer screenings. Continue to take all medicines as prescribed.

Your preferences about treatment are always important. Talk to your care team and make your wishes known.

8
Recurrence

77 Overview

77 Tests

77 Treatment

79 Key points

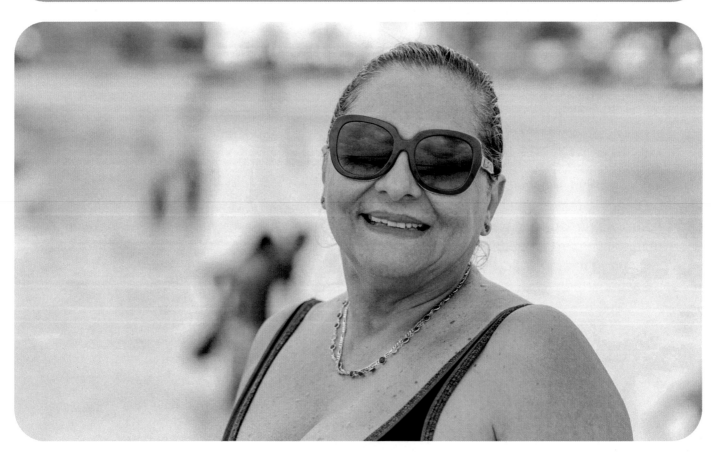

When cancer returns, it is called a recurrence. Treatment is based on the types of treatment you had before. Together, you and your doctor will choose a treatment plan that is best for you.

Overview

Breast cancer can return in 3 places:

> It can return to the breast that had cancer before. This is called a local recurrence.

> It can return to axillary lymph nodes or lymph nodes in or near the breast. This is called a regional occurrence.

> It can return in other distant parts of the body. This is called metastatic breast cancer.

This chapter presents treatment options for local and regional recurrence.

When breast cancer has spread to distant parts of the body, it is called metastatic breast cancer.

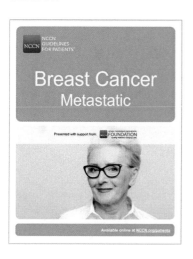

For more information, read the *NCCN Guidelines for Patients: Breast Cancer – Metastatic,* available at NCCN.org/ patientguidelines.

Tests

You will have tests to learn more about your cancer. Many tests you had when you were first diagnosed will be repeated. This is called restaging. Tests such as a brain or spine MRI might be done based on your symptoms. Tests for recurrence can be found in Guide 13.

Treatment

Treatment is based on where the cancer has returned and what type of treatment you had before. Surgery followed by radiation therapy (RT) and systemic therapy are possible. Systemic and endocrine therapy options will be based on tumor hormone receptor (HR) status, HER2 status, and previous treatments given during your initial cancer treatment. Supportive care will be given. Supportive care aims to relieve side effects such as pain and to improve quality of life.

Local only
Treatment for a local recurrence is based on if your first treatment was breast-conserving surgery (lumpectomy) with radiation therapy or a mastectomy with or without radiation therapy (RT). More surgery might be an option. However, if you had RT before, then it may not be possible to have it again in the same area.

Regional only
If the regional recurrence is in or near the armpit (axilla), then surgery to remove the tumor might be an option before RT. Systemic therapy might be given before surgery to help reduce the disease burden.

Both local and regional

Cancer that is both local and regional might be referred to as a locoregional recurrence. Treatment for a locoregional recurrence is surgery and RT when possible. Some people receive systemic therapy or RT if surgery is not possible.

Unresectable

An unresectable tumor cannot be removed with surgery. It is treated with systemic therapy. For treatment of unresectable recurrent disease, see NCCN Guidelines for Patients: Breast Cancer – Metastatic, available at NCCN.org/patientguidelines.

Guide 13
Possible tests: Recurrence

Medical history and physical exam

Discuss goals of therapy, engage in shared decision-making, and document course of care

CBC and comprehensive metabolic panel (including liver function tests and alkaline phosphatase)

Diagnostic chest CT with or without contrast

CT with contrast of abdomen with or without pelvis (MRI with contrast might be done instead)

Brain MRI with contrast if suspicious central nervous system (CNS) symptoms

Spine MRI with contrast if back pain or symptoms of cord compression

Bone scan or sodium fluoride PET/CT, if needed

FDG PET/CT, as needed

X-rays of symptomatic bones and long and weight-bearing bones abnormal on bone scan

Biopsy tumor or metastasis and test for biomarkers

Determine tumor status including:
- Estrogen receptor (ER) and progesterone receptor (PR) hormone receptor (HR) status
- HER2 status

Genetic counseling if at risk for hereditary breast cancer

Assess for distress

Key points

> When cancer returns, it is called a recurrence.

> Cancer that returns to the breast that had cancer before is called a local recurrence.

> Cancer that returns to axillary lymph nodes or lymph nodes in or near the breast is called a regional recurrence.

> Cancer that returns in distant parts of the body is called metastatic breast cancer.

> Treatment is based on where the cancer has returned and what type of treatment you had before.

> Surgery followed by radiation therapy and systemic therapy are possible. Systemic and endocrine therapy options will be based on hormone receptor and HER2 status, and any mutations found.

> Supportive care will be given. Supportive care aims to relieve side effects such as pain and to improve quality of life.

> An unresectable tumor cannot be removed with surgery. Unresectable recurrent disease is treated as metastatic disease with systemic therapy.

> More information on recurrence can be found in *NCCN Guidelines for Patients: Breast Cancer – Metastatic,* available at NCCN.org/patientguidelines.

Supportive care aims to prevent, reduce, and relieve side effects and to improve quality of life.

9

Inflammatory breast cancer

81 Overview

81 Tests

83 Treatment

84 Treatment response

87 Key points

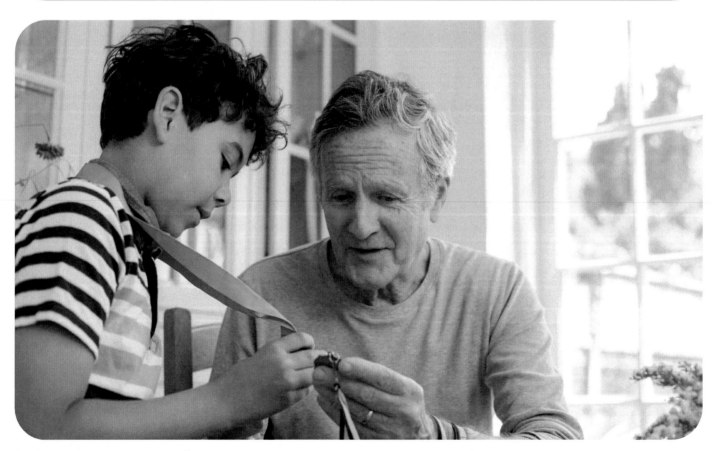

Inflammatory breast cancer (IBC) is a rare, aggressive cancer where cancer cells block lymph vessels in the skin of the breast. This causes the breast to look red and swollen and feel warm to the touch. Treatment is systemic therapy to shrink the tumor, followed by surgery to remove the breast and lymph nodes, and then radiation. Together, you and your doctor will choose a treatment plan that is best for you.

Overview

Most inflammatory breast cancers (IBCs) are invasive ductal carcinomas. This means that cancer started in the cells that line the milk ducts and has spread into surrounding tissue. At diagnosis, IBC is stage 3 or 4 disease. In stage 3, cancer may be in nearby lymph nodes. In stage 4, cancer is in nearby lymph nodes and has spread to other parts of the body (metastasized).

Since IBC spreads quickly, treatment starts with systemic therapy to stop the spread of cancer. If the cancer responds to treatment, then surgery to remove the breast and lymph nodes (modified radical mastectomy) will be done. This is followed with radiation to the chest wall. If you want breast reconstruction after a mastectomy with radiation, then delayed breast reconstruction is an option. Radiation can slow the healing process. Therefore, reconstruction is recommended after all the healing from radiation is done.

Like other breast cancers, IBC can happen in those assigned male at birth.

Tests

IBC can be difficult to diagnose. Often, there is no lump that can be felt during a breast exam or seen on a mammogram. Since there is swelling and redness of the breast, IBC can look like an infection and therefore be difficult to diagnose. Often, a biopsy of the affected skin is done to diagnose the tumor.

You will have blood tests, imaging tests, and a tumor biopsy to stage the cancer. The biopsy sample will be tested for hormone receptors (estrogen and progesterone) and HER2 receptors. Treatment will be based on these findings.

Imaging and staging tests may include the following:

> ⟩ A bilateral diagnostic mammogram and an ultrasound of the breast and regional (nearby) lymph nodes

> ⟩ A CT, MRI, or a PET/CT scan and a bone scan to see if the cancer has spread to other parts of the body before starting any treatments

Tests for IBC can be found in Guide 14.

Guide 14
Possible tests: Inflammatory breast cancer (IBC)

Medical history and physical exam by multidisciplinary team

CBC and comprehensive metabolic panel (including liver function tests and alkaline phosphatase)

Biopsy with pathology review

Determine tumor status including:
- Estrogen receptor (ER) and progesterone receptor (PR) hormone receptor (HR) status
- HER2 status

Fertility counseling if premenopausal

Genetic counseling if at risk for hereditary breast cancer

Bilateral diagnostic mammogram

Ultrasound as needed

Chest CT with or without contrast

CT with contrast of abdomen with or without pelvis (MRI with contrast might be done instead)

Bone scan or FDG-PET/CT

Breast MRI, if needed

Treatment

Treatment for IBC starts with preoperative systemic therapy. Preoperative therapy is treatment given before surgery. It is based on if the tumor is HER2-positive (HER2+) or HER2-negative (HER2-).

HER2-

For HER2- cancer, the preferred treatment is an anthracycline with a taxane. These are types of chemotherapy. Anthracyclines include doxorubicin and epirubicin. Docetaxel, paclitaxel, and albumin-bound paclitaxel are taxanes.

HER2+

IBCs often produce greater than normal amounts of HER2. If the tumor is HER2+, then HER2-targeted therapy should be given as preoperative systemic therapy. Systemic therapy options for HER2+ can be found in Guide 15.

Guide 15 Systemic therapy options: HER2+	
Preferred options	• Paclitaxel and trastuzumab • Docetaxel, carboplatin, and trastuzumab (TCH) • Docetaxel, carboplatin, trastuzumab, and pertuzumab (TCHP) • Complete up to one year of HER2-targeted therapy with trastuzumab. Pertuzumab might be added
Other recommended	• Doxorubicin with cyclophosphamide followed by docetaxel with trastuzumab • Doxorubicin with cyclophosphamide followed by docetaxel with trastuzumab and pertuzumab
Used in some cases	• Docetaxel, cyclophosphamide, and trastuzumab • Doxorubicin and cyclophosphamide followed by paciltaxel with trastuzumab • Doxorubicin and cyclophosphamide followed by docetaxel with paclitaxel, trastuzumab, and pertuzumab • Neratinib • Paclitaxel with trastuzumab and pertuzumab • Ado-trastuzumab emtansine (TDM-1)

Note: An FDA-approved biosimilar might be used for trastuzumab.

Treatment response

The next treatment is based on how the tumor responded to preoperative systemic therapy. It is called preoperative (before surgery) treatment because the goal is surgery, when possible. Systemic treatment after surgery is called adjuvant therapy.

A physical exam and imaging tests should be done to assess how the cancer responded to preoperative systemic therapy. Treatment will be based on if the tumor shrunk and surgery is possible or if the tumor did not shrink enough to be removed with surgery.

Guide 16 Adjuvant endocrine therapy		
Premenopause at diagnosis	• Tamoxifen alone for 5 years • Tamoxifen for 5 years with ovarian suppression or ablation →	• After 5 years, if in postmenopause, then an aromatase inhibitor for 5 years or consider tamoxifen for another 5 years (for a total of 10 years on tamoxifen) • After 5 years, if still in premenopause, then consider tamoxifen for another 5 years (for a total of 10 years on tamoxifen) or stop endocrine therapy
	• Aromatase inhibitor for 5 years with ovarian suppression or ablation. Then consider aromatase inhibitor for an additional 3 to 5 years	
Menopause at diagnosis	• Aromatase inhibitor for 5 years, then consider aromatase inhibitor for 3 to 5 more years • Aromatase inhibitor for 2 to 3 years, then tamoxifen to complete 5 years total of endocrine therapy • Tamoxifen for 2 to 3 years, then an aromatase inhibitor to complete 5 years of endocrine therapy • Tamoxifen for 2 to 3 years, then up to 5 years of an aromatase inhibitor	
	• Tamoxifen for 4.5 to 6 years, then an aromatase inhibitor for 5 years or consider tamoxifen for another 5 years (for a total of 10 years on tamoxifen)	
	• For those who can't have aromatase inhibitors or who don't want aromatase inhibitors, take tamoxifen for 5 years or consider tamoxifen for up to 10 years	

Surgery is an option

If the tumor shrunk enough so surgery is possible, then a total mastectomy with level I and II axillary lymph node dissection is the recommended option. You may choose a delayed breast reconstruction as part of the mastectomy. Radiation therapy (RT) is part of this treatment.

After the mastectomy and RT, you will finish chemotherapy if you didn't complete the course before surgery. If the tumor is ER+ and/or PR+, then you will have endocrine therapy. Endocrine therapy is used to treat tumors that are estrogen receptor-positive (ER+) and/or progesterone receptor-positive (PR+).

If the tumor is HER2+, then you will have up to one year of HER2-targeted therapy. This may be given with RT and endocrine therapy.

For a list of systemic therapies that target HER2+, see Guide 15.

For a list of adjuvant endocrine therapy options, see Guide 16.

Surgery is not an option

Surgery is not always possible. Even though surgery might not be an option, systemic therapy will continue. If the cancer is not responding to systemic therapy, then radiation may be considered to try to make the cancer resectable (able to be removed with surgery). The goal of treatment is to reduce the amount of cancer. Talk with your doctor about your goals of treatment and your treatment preferences. Your wishes are always important.

For a list of systemic therapies that target HER2+, see Guide 15.

For a list of systemic therapies for HER2-, see Guide 17.

Guide 17
Systemic therapy options: HER2-

Preferred options	• Doxorubicin and cyclophosphamide followed by paclitaxel • Docetaxel and cyclophosphamide (TC) • Olaparib, if germline *BRCA1* or *BRCA2* mutations
	• High-risk triple-negative breast cancer (TNBC): Preoperative pembrolizumab with carboplatin and paclitaxel, followed by preoperative pembrolizumab and cyclophosphamide with doxorubicin or epirubicin, followed by adjuvant pembrolizumab • If TNBC and residual disease after preoperative therapy with taxane-, alkylator-, and anthracycline-based chemotherapy, then capecitabine
Other recommended	• Doxorubicin and cyclophosphamide followed by docetaxel • Epirubicin and cyclophosphamide (EC) • Docetaxel, doxorubicin, and cyclophosphamide (TAC)
	Only in certain TNBC cases: • Paclitaxel with carboplatin • Docetaxel with carboplatin (preoperative setting only)
Used in some cases	• Doxorubicin and cyclophosphamide • Cyclophosphamide, methotrexate, and fluorouracil (CMF) • Doxorubicin and cyclophosphamide followed by paclitaxel • Capecitabine (maintenance therapy for TNBC after adjuvant chemotherapy)

Key points

- In inflammatory breast cancer (IBC), cancer cells block lymph vessels in the skin of the breast. This causes the breast to look red and swollen and feel warm to the touch.

- IBC is treated with systemic therapy to shrink the tumor, followed by surgery to remove the tumor, and then radiation therapy. Surgery is not always possible. Even though surgery might not be an option, systemic therapy will continue.

- Treatment is based on blood tests, imaging tests, and a biopsy to stage the cancer. The biopsy sample will be tested for hormone receptors and HER2 receptors.

- IBCs often produce greater than normal amounts of HER2. If the tumor is HER2+, then HER2-targeted therapy may be given as preoperative systemic therapy.

- Endocrine therapy is used to treat tumors that are estrogen receptor-positive (ER+) and/or progesterone receptor-positive (PR+).

- Systemic therapy given after surgery is called adjuvant therapy. Adjuvant systemic therapy may be given after surgery to reduce the chance of cancer recurrence.

Need help paying for medicine or treatment?

Ask your care team what options are available.

10
Making treatment decisions

89   It's your choice

89   Questions to ask your doctors

98   Resources

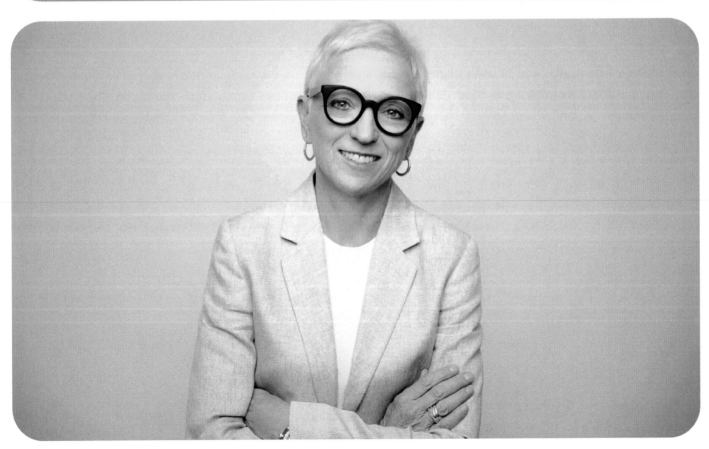

It's important to be comfortable with the cancer treatment you choose. This choice starts with having an open and honest conversation with your doctor.

It's your choice

In shared decision-making, you and your doctors share information, discuss the options, and agree on a treatment plan. It starts with an open and honest conversation between you and your doctor.

Treatment decisions are very personal. What is important to you may not be important to someone else.

Some things that may play a role in your decision-making:

> What you want and how that might differ from what others want

> Your religious and spiritual beliefs

> Your feelings about certain treatments like surgery or chemotherapy

> Your feelings about pain or side effects such as nausea and vomiting

> Cost of treatment, travel to treatment centers, and time away from school or work

> Quality of life and length of life

> How active you are and the activities that are important to you

Think about what you want from treatment. Discuss openly the risks and benefits of specific treatments and procedures. Weigh options and share concerns with your doctor. If you take the time to build a relationship with your doctor, it will help you feel supported when considering options and making treatment decisions.

Second opinion

It is normal to want to start treatment as soon as possible. While cancer can't be ignored, there is time to have another doctor review your test results and suggest a treatment plan. This is called getting a second opinion, and it's a normal part of cancer care. Even doctors get second opinions!

Things you can do to prepare:

> Check with your insurance company about its rules on second opinions. There may be out-of-pocket costs to see doctors who are not part of your insurance plan.

> Make plans to have copies of all your records sent to the doctor you will see for your second opinion.

Support groups

Many people diagnosed with cancer find support groups to be helpful. Support groups often include people at different stages of treatment. Some people may be newly diagnosed, while others may be finished with treatment. If your hospital or community doesn't have support groups for people with cancer, check out the websites listed in this book.

Questions to ask your doctors

Possible questions to ask your doctors are listed on the following pages. Feel free to use these questions or come up with your own. Be clear about your goals for treatment and find out what to expect from treatment.

Questions to ask about testing and diagnosis

1. What tests will I have? How often will they be repeated? Will my insurance pay for these tests?

2. What will you do to make me comfortable during testing?

3. What if I am pregnant or want to become pregnant?

4. When will I have a biopsy? Will I have more than one? What are the risks?

5. How will my biopsy be performed? What else might be done at this time?

6. How soon will I know the results and who will explain them to me?

7. How can I get a copy of the pathology report and other test results?

8. Who will talk with me about the next steps? When?

9. What can I do before my next appointment?

Questions to ask your care team about their experience

1. What is your experience treating this type cancer?

2. What is the experience of those on your team?

3. Do you only treat invasive breast cancer? What else do you treat?

4. How many patients like me (of the same age, gender, race) have you treated?

5. Will you be consulting with experts to discuss my care? Whom will you consult?

6. How many procedures like the one you're suggesting have you done?

7. Is this treatment a major part of your practice?

8. How many of your patients have had complications? What were the complications?

9. How many breast cancer surgeries have you done? What type of surgeries have you done? How many per year?

10. Who will manage my day-to-day care?

Questions to ask about options

1. What will happen if I do nothing?

2. How do my age, overall health, and other factors affect my options?

3. What if I am pregnant? What if I'm planning to get pregnant in the near future?

4. Which option is proven to work best for my cancer, age, and other risk factors?

5. What are the possible complications and side effects?

6. How do you know if the treatment worked? How will I know?

7. What can be done to prevent or relieve the side effects of treatment?

8. Are there any life-threatening side effects of this treatment? How will I be monitored?

9. Am I a candidate for a clinical trial? Can I join a clinical trial at any time?

10. Does any option offer a long-term cancer control? Are the chances any better for one option than another? Less time-consuming? Less expensive?

11. Is there a social worker or someone who can help me decide?

12. Is there a hospital or treatment center you can recommend for breast cancer treatment? Can I go to one hospital for surgery and a different center for radiation therapy?

Questions to ask about treatment

1. What are my treatment choices? What are the benefits and risks? Which treatment do you recommend and why?

2. How will my age, performance status, cancer stage, and other health conditions limit my treatment choices?

3. Does the order of treatment matter?

4. How long do I have to decide about treatment?

5. Will I have to go to the hospital or elsewhere for treatment? How often? How long is each visit? Will I have to stay overnight in the hospital or make travel plans?

6. Do I have a choice of when to begin treatment? Can I choose the days and times of treatment? Should I bring someone with me?

7. How much will the treatment hurt? What will you do to make me comfortable?

8. Can I stop treatment at any time? What will happen if I stop treatment?

9. How much will this treatment cost me? How much will my insurance pay for this treatment? Are there any programs to help me pay for treatment?

10. Will I miss work or school? Will I be able to drive? When will I be able to return to my normal activities?

11. What are the chances my cancer will return after this treatment? How will it be treated if it returns?

12. I would like a second opinion. Is there someone you can recommend? Who can help me gather all of my records for a second opinion?

Questions to ask about surgery

1. How much of my breast will be removed? What will it look like afterwards?

2. What other organs or tissues might be removed during surgery? What will this mean in terms of my recovery?

3. What kind of surgery will I have? Will I have more than one surgery?

4. What are the chances you can remove the whole tumor and I will have a negative margin?

5. How long will it take me to recover from surgery? When will I be able to return to work?

6. How much pain will I be in? What will be done to manage my pain?

7. What is the chance that this surgery will shorten my life?

8. What other side effects can I expect from surgery? What complications can occur from this surgery?

9. What treatment will I have before, during, or after surgery? What does this treatment do?

10. I am considering a mastectomy with flat closure. Can you tell me more about this procedure?

11. I am considering a mastectomy with reconstruction. Can you tell me about the options?

Questions to ask about radiation therapy

1. What type of radiation therapy (RT) will I have?

2. What will you target?

3. What is the goal of this RT?

4. How many treatment sessions will I require? Can you do a shorter course of RT?

5. Do you offer this type of RT here? If not, can you refer me to someone who does?

6. What side effects can I expect from RT?

7. Should I eat or drink before RT?

8. Will I be given medicine to help me relax during RT?

9. What should I wear?

Questions to ask about side effects

1. What are the side effects of treatment?

2. What are the side effects of this cancer?

3. How long will these side effects last? Do any side effects lessen or worsen in severity over time?

4. What side effects should I watch for? What side effects are expected and which are life threatening?

5. When should I call the doctor? Can I text? What should I do on weekends and during non-office hours?

6. What emergency department or ER should I go to? Will my treatment team be able to communicate with the ER team?

7. What medicines can I take to prevent or relieve side effects?

8. What can I do to help with pain and other side effects?

9. Will you stop treatment or change treatment if there are side effects? What do you look for?

10. What can I do to lessen or prevent side effects? What will you do?

11. What medicines may worsen side effects of treatment?

12. What are some of the likely permanent side effects that I might have from the treatment?

Questions to ask about clinical trials

1. What clinical trials are available for my type and stage of breast cancer?

2. What are the treatments used in the clinical trial?

3. What does the treatment do?

4. Has the treatment been used before? Has it been used for other types of cancer?

5. What are the risks and benefits of this treatment?

6. What side effects should I expect? How will the side effects be controlled?

7. How long will I be in the clinical trial?

8. Will I be able to get other treatments if this doesn't work?

9. How will you know the treatment is working?

10. Will the clinical trial cost me anything? If so, how much?

11. How do I find out about clinical trials that I can participate in? Are there online sources that I can search?

Resources

American Association for Cancer Research (AACR)
aacr.org

American Breast Cancer Foundation
youandbreastcancer.com/en-bc/home

American Cancer Society (ACS)
cancer.org/cancer/breast-cancer.html

American Society of Clinical Oncology (ASCO)
cancer.net

Breast Cancer Alliance (BCA)
breastcanceralliance.org

Breast Cancer Support Project
breastcancerportraitproject.org

Breastcancer.org
breastcancer.org

Brem Foundation
bremfoundation.org

Cancer*Care*
cancercare.org

Cancer Support Community
cancersupportcommunity.org/living-cancer

Chemocare
chemocare.com

DiepCFoundation
diepcfoundation.org

FORCE - Facing Our Risk of Cancer Empowered
facingourrisk.org

GPAC - Global Patient Advocacy Coalition
GPACunited.org

Healthwell Foundation
healthwellfoundation.org

Inflammatory Breast Cancer Research Foundation
ibcresearch.org

Living Beyond Breast Cancer (LBBC)
lbbc.org

MedlinePlus
medlineplus.gov/breastcancer.html

My Survival Story
mysurvivalstory.org

National Cancer Institute (NCI)
cancer.gov/types/breast

National Center for Health Research
breastimplantinfo.org

National Coalition for Cancer Survivorship
canceradvocacy.org/toolbox

National Financial Resource Directory - Patient Advocate Foundation
patientadvocate.org/explore-our-resources/national-financial-resource-directory/

OncoLink
oncolink.org

Patient Access Network Foundation
panfoundation.org

Radiological Society of North America
radiologyinfo.org

SHARE Cancer Support
sharecancersupport.org

Sharsheret
sharsheret.org

Smart Patients
smartpatients.com/communities/breast-cancer

Susan G. Komen
komen.org

Testing.com
testing.com

The Male Breast Cancer Coalition
malebreastcancercoalition.org/men-have-breasts-too

Unite for HER
uniteforher.org

Young Survival Coalition (YSC)
youngsurvival.org

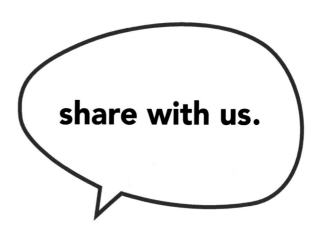

Take our survey
And help make the
NCCN Guidelines for Patients
better for everyone!

NCCN.org/patients/comments

Words to know

accelerated partial breast irradiation (APBI)
Treatment with radiation of part of the breast with cancer. A higher dose is given over a shorter period of time compared to whole breast radiation therapy.

adjuvant therapy
Treatment that is given to lower the chances of the cancer returning.

anti-estrogen
A cancer drug that stops estrogen from attaching to cells.

areola
A darker, round area of skin on the breast around the nipple.

aromatase inhibitor (AI)
A drug that lowers the level of estrogen in the body.

axillary lymph node (ALN)
A small disease-fighting structure that is near the armpit.

axillary lymph node dissection (ALND)
An operation that removes the disease-fighting structures (lymph nodes) near the armpit.

bilateral diagnostic mammogram
Pictures of the insides of both breasts that are made from a set of x-rays.

bilateral oophorectomy
An operation that removes both ovaries.

biopsy
A procedure that removes fluid or tissue samples to be tested for a disease.

bone mineral density
A test that measures the strength of bones.

bone scan
A test that makes pictures of bones to assess for health problems.

boost
An extra dose of radiation to a specific area of the body.

breast-conserving surgery (BCS)
A cancer treatment that includes removing a breast lump.

breast implant
A small bag filled with salt water, gel, or both that is used to remake breasts.

breast reconstruction
An operation that creates new breasts.

cancer stage
A rating of the outlook of a cancer based on its growth and spread.

carcinoma
A cancer of cells that line the inner or outer surfaces of the body.

chemotherapy
Cancer drugs that stop the cell life cycle so cells don't increase in number.

chest wall
The layer of muscle, bone, and fat that protects the vital organs.

clinical breast exam
Touching of a breast by a health expert to feel for diseases.

clinical stage (c)
The rating of the extent of cancer before treatment is started.

clinical trial
A type of research that assesses health tests or treatments.

complete blood count (CBC)
A lab test that includes the number of blood cells.

computed tomography (CT)
A test that uses x-rays from many angles to make a picture of the insides of the body.

connective tissue
Supporting and binding tissue that surrounds other tissues and organs.

contrast
A substance put into your body to make clearer pictures during imaging tests.

core needle biopsy
A procedure that removes tissue samples with a hollow needle. Also called core biopsy.

deoxyribonucleic acid (DNA)
A chain of chemicals in cells that contains coded instructions for making and controlling cells.

diagnostic bilateral mammogram
Pictures of the insides of both breasts that are made from a set of x-rays.

duct
A tube-shaped structure through which milk travels to the nipple.

ductal carcinoma
A cancer derived from cells that line small tube-shaped vessels.

endocrine therapy
A cancer treatment that stops the making or action of estrogen. Also called hormone therapy.

estrogen
A hormone that causes female body traits.

estrogen receptor (ER)
A protein inside of cells that binds to estrogen.

estrogen receptor-negative (ER-)
A type of breast cancer that doesn't use estrogen to grow.

estrogen receptor-positive (ER+)
A type of breast cancer that uses estrogen to grow.

fertility specialist
An expert who helps people to have babies.

fine-needle aspiration (FNA)
A procedure that removes tissue samples with a very thin needle.

flat closure
Procedure done after a mastectomy in which the skin is tightened and sewn together without the addition of a breast implant.

gene
Coded instructions in cells for making new cells and controlling how cells behave.

genetic counseling
Expert guidance on the chance for a disease that is passed down in families.

hereditary breast cancer
Breast cancer that was likely caused by abnormal genes passed down from parent to child.

histology
The structure of cells, tissue, and organs as viewed under a microscope.

hormone
A chemical in the body that triggers a response from cells or organs.

hormone receptor-negative cancer (HR-)
Cancer cells that don't use hormones to grow.

hormone receptor-positive cancer (HR+)
Cancer cells that use hormones to grow.

human epidermal growth factor receptor 2 (HER2)
A protein on the edge of a cell that sends signals for the cell to grow.

imaging test
A test that makes pictures (images) of the insides of the body.

immune system
The body's natural defense against infection and disease.

immunohistochemistry (IHC)
A lab test of cancer cells to find specific cell traits involved in abnormal cell growth.

in situ hybridization (ISH)
A lab test of the number of a gene.

inflammatory breast cancer
A type of breast cancer in which the breast looks red and swollen and feels warm to the touch.

infraclavicular
The area right below the collarbone.

internal mammary
The area along the breastbone.

invasive breast cancer
The growth of breast cancer into the breast's supporting tissue (stroma).

lobule
A gland in the breast that makes breast milk.

lobular carcinoma
A breast cancer that started in cells that line the breast glands (lobules).

lumpectomy
An operation that removes a small breast cancer tumor. Also called breast-conserving surgery.

luteinizing hormone-releasing hormone (LHRH)
A hormone in the brain that helps control the making of estrogen by the ovaries.

lymph
A clear fluid containing white blood cells.

lymph node
A small, bean-shaped disease-fighting structure.

lymphadenopathy
Lymph nodes that are abnormal in size or consistency.

lymphatic system
Germ-fighting network of tissues and organs that includes the bone marrow, spleen, thymus, lymph nodes, and lymphatic vessels. Part of the immune system.

lymphedema
Swelling in the body due to a buildup of fluid called lymph.

magnetic resonance imaging (MRI)
A test that uses radio waves and powerful magnets to make pictures of the insides of the body.

mammogram
A picture of the insides of the breast that is made by an x-ray test.

mastectomy
An operation that removes the whole breast.

medical history
A report of all your health events and medications.

medical oncologist
A doctor who is an expert in cancer drugs.

menopause
The point in time 12 months after a last menstrual period.

mutation
An abnormal change.

neoadjuvant treatment
A treatment that is given before the main treatment to reduce the cancer. Also called preoperative treatment if given before an operation.

nipple-areola complex (NAC)
The ring of darker breast skin is called the areola. The raised tip within the areola is called the nipple.

noninvasive breast cancer
Breast cancer that has not grown into tissue from which it can spread.

ovarian ablation
Methods used to stop the ovaries from making hormones.

ovarian suppression
A drug treatment that lowers the amount of hormones made by the ovaries.

palpable adenopathy
Lymph nodes that feel abnormal in size or consistency.

partial breast irradiation
Treatment with radiation that is received at the site of the removed breast tumor.

pathologic stage (p)
A rating of the extent of cancer based on tests given after treatment.

pathologist
A doctor who's an expert in testing cells and tissue to find disease.

pelvis
The body area between the hip bones.

physical exam
A study of the body by a health expert for signs of disease.

positron emission tomography (PET)
A test that uses radioactive material to see the shape and function of body parts.

postmenopause
The state of having no more menstrual periods.

premenopause
The state of having menstrual periods.

primary tumor
The first mass of cancer cells.

progesterone
A hormone in women that is involved in sexual development, periods, and pregnancy.

prognosis
The likely course and outcome of a disease based on tests.

radiation therapy (RT)
A treatment that uses high-energy rays.

recurrence
The return of cancer after a cancer-free period.

selective estrogen receptor degrader (SERD)
A drug that blocks and destroys estrogen receptors.

selective estrogen receptor modulator (SERM)
A drug that blocks the effect of estrogen inside of cells.

sentinel lymph node (SLN)
The first lymph node to which cancer cells spread after leaving a tumor.

sentinel lymph node biopsy (SLNB)
An operation to remove the disease-fighting structures (lymph nodes) to which cancer first spreads. Also called sentinel lymph node dissection.

side effect
An unhealthy or unpleasant physical or emotional response to treatment.

skin-sparing mastectomy
An operation that removes all breast tissue but saves as much breast skin as possible.

supportive care
Health care that includes symptom relief but not cancer treatment. Also called palliative care or best supportive care.

supraclavicular
The area right above the collarbone.

surgical margin
The normal-looking tissue around a tumor that was removed during an operation.

systemic therapy
Drug treatment that works throughout the body.

total mastectomy
An operation that removes the entire breast but no chest muscles. Also called simple mastectomy.

triple-negative breast cancer (TNBC)
A breast cancer that does not use hormones or the HER2 protein to grow.

ultrasound
A test that uses sound waves to take pictures of the inside of the body.

volume displacement
A method to shift breast tissue during an operation to fill a gap.

vulva
The outer female organs that are between the legs.

whole breast radiation therapy (WBRT)
Treatment with radiation of the entire breast.

NCCN Contributors

This patient guide is based on the for The NCCN Clinical Practice Guidelines in Oncology (NCCN Guidelines®) for Breast Cancer, Version 2.2022. It was adapted, reviewed, and published with help from the following people:

Dorothy A. Shead, MS
Senior Director
Patient Information Operations

Tanya Fischer, MEd, MSLIS
Medical Writer

Susan Kidney
Senior Graphic Design Specialist

The NCCN Clinical Practice Guidelines in Oncology (NCCN Guidelines®) for Breast Cancer, Version 2.2022 were developed by the following NCCN Panel Members:

William J. Gradishar, MD/Chair
Robert H. Lurie Comprehensive Cancer Center of Northwestern University

Meena S. Moran, MD/Vice-Chair
Yale Cancer Center/Smilow Cancer Hospital

Jame Abraham, MD
Case Comprehensive Cancer Center/ University Hospitals Seidman Cancer Center and Cleveland Clinic Taussig Cancer Institute

Rebecca Aft, MD, PhD
Siteman Cancer Center at Barnes-Jewish Hospital and Washington University School of Medicine

*Doreen Agnese, MD
The Ohio State University Comprehensive Cancer Center - James Cancer Hospital and Solove Research Institute

Kimberly H. Allison, MD
Stanford Cancer Institute

Bethany Anderson, MD
University of Wisconsin Carbone Cancer Center

Sarah L. Blair, MD
UC San Diego Moores Cancer Center

Harold J. Burstein, MD, PhD
Dana-Farber/Brigham and Women's Cancer Center

Helen Chew, MD
UC Davis Comprehensive Cancer Center

Chau Dang, MD
Memorial Sloan Kettering Cancer Center

Anthony D. Elias, MD
University of Colorado Cancer Center

Sharon H. Giordano, MD, MPH
The University of Texas MD Anderson Cancer Center

Matthew Goetz, MD
Mayo Clinic Cancer Center

Lori J. Goldstein, MD
Fox Chase Cancer Center

Sara A. Hurvitz, MD
UCLA Jonsson Comprehensive Cancer Center

Steven J. Isakoff, MD, PhD
Massachusetts General Hospital Cancer Center

Rachel C. Jankowitz, MD
Abramson Cancer Center at the University of Pennsylvania

Sara H. Javid, MD
Fred Hutchinson Cancer Research Center/Seattle Cancer Care Alliance

Jairam Krishnamurthy, MD
Fred & Pamela Buffet Cancer Center

Marilyn Leitch, MD
UT Southwestern Simmons Comprehensive Cancer Center

Janice Lyons, MD
Case Comprehensive Cancer Center/ University Hospitals Seidman Cancer Center and Cleveland Clinic Taussig Cancer Institute

Ingrid A. Mayer, MD
Vanderbilt-Ingram Cancer Center

Joanne Mortimer, MD
City of Hope National Medical Center

Sameer A. Patel, MD
Fox Chase Cancer Center

Lori J. Pierce, MD
University of Michigan Rogel Cancer Center

Laura H. Rosenberger, MD, MS
Duke Cancer Institute

Hope S. Rugo, MD
UCSF Helen Diller Family Comprehensive Cancer Center

*Amy Sitapati, MD
UC San Diego Moores Cancer Center

Karen Lisa Smith, MD, MPH
The Sidney Kimmel Comprehensive Cancer Center at Johns Hopkins

Mary Lou Smith, JD, MBA
Patient Advocate Research Advocacy Network

Hatem Soliman, MD
Moffitt Cancer Center

Erica M. Stringer-Reasor, MD
O'Neal Comprehensive Cancer Center at UAB

Melinda L. Telli, MD
Stanford Cancer Institute

John H. Ward, MD
Huntsman Cancer Institute at the University of Utah

Kari B. Wisinski, MD
University of Wisconsin Carbone Cancer Center

*Jessica S. Young, MD
Roswell Park Comprehensive Cancer Center

NCCN Staff

Rashmi Kumar, PhD
Director, Clinical Information Operations

Jennifer Burns, BS
Manager, Guidelines Support

* Reviewed this patient guide. For disclosures, visit NCCN.org/disclosures.

NCCN Cancer Centers

Abramson Cancer Center
at the University of Pennsylvania
Philadelphia, Pennsylvania
800.789.7366 • pennmedicine.org/cancer

Case Comprehensive Cancer Center/
University Hospitals Seidman Cancer
Center and Cleveland Clinic Taussig
Cancer Institute
Cleveland, Ohio
800.641.2422 • UH Seidman Cancer Center
uhhospitals.org/services/cancer-services
866.223.8100 • CC Taussig Cancer Institute
my.clevelandclinic.org/departments/cancer
216.844.8797 • Case CCC
case.edu/cancer

City of Hope National Medical Center
Los Angeles, California
800.826.4673 • cityofhope.org

Dana-Farber/Brigham and Women's
Cancer Center | Massachusetts General
Hospital Cancer Center
Boston, Massachusetts
617.732.5500 • youhaveus.org
617.726.5130
massgeneral.org/cancer-center

Duke Cancer Institute
Durham, North Carolina
888.275.3853 • dukecancerinstitute.org

Fox Chase Cancer Center
Philadelphia, Pennsylvania
888.369.2427 • foxchase.org

Fred & Pamela Buffett Cancer Center
Omaha, Nebraska
402.559.5600 • unmc.edu/cancercenter

Fred Hutchinson Cancer
Research Center/Seattle
Cancer Care Alliance
Seattle, Washington
206.606.7222 • seattlecca.org
206.667.5000 • fredhutch.org

Huntsman Cancer Institute
at the University of Utah
Salt Lake City, Utah
800.824.2073 • huntsmancancer.org

Indiana University
Melvin and Bren Simon
Comprehensive Cancer Center
Indianapolis, Indiana
www.cancer.iu.edu

Mayo Clinic Cancer Center
Phoenix/Scottsdale, Arizona
Jacksonville, Florida
Rochester, Minnesota
480.301.8000 • Arizona
904.953.0853 • Florida
507.538.3270 • Minnesota
mayoclinic.org/cancercenter

Memorial Sloan Kettering
Cancer Center
New York, New York
800.525.2225 • mskcc.org

Moffitt Cancer Center
Tampa, Florida
888.663.3488 • moffitt.org

O'Neal Comprehensive
Cancer Center at UAB
Birmingham, Alabama
800.822.0933 • uab.edu/onealcancercenter

Robert H. Lurie Comprehensive Cancer
Center of Northwestern University
Chicago, Illinois
866.587.4322 • cancer.northwestern.edu

Roswell Park Comprehensive
Cancer Center
Buffalo, New York
877.275.7724 • roswellpark.org

Siteman Cancer Center at Barnes-
Jewish Hospital and Washington
University School of Medicine
St. Louis, Missouri
800.600.3606 • siteman.wustl.edu

St. Jude Children's
Research Hospital/
The University of Tennessee
Health Science Center
Memphis, Tennessee
866.278.5833 • stjude.org
901.448.5500 • uthsc.edu

Stanford Cancer Institute
Stanford, California
877.668.7535 • cancer.stanford.edu

The Ohio State University
Comprehensive Cancer Center -
James Cancer Hospital and
Solove Research Institute
Columbus, Ohio
800.293.5066 • cancer.osu.edu

The Sidney Kimmel Comprehensive
Cancer Center at Johns Hopkins
Baltimore, Maryland
410.955.8964
www.hopkinskimmelcancercenter.org

The University of Texas
MD Anderson Cancer Center
Houston, Texas
844.269.5922 • mdanderson.org

UC Davis
Comprehensive Cancer Center
Sacramento, California
916.734.5959 • 800.770.9261
health.ucdavis.edu/cancer

UC San Diego Moores Cancer Center
La Jolla, California
858.822.6100 • cancer.ucsd.edu

UCLA Jonsson
Comprehensive Cancer Center
Los Angeles, California
310.825.5268 • cancer.ucla.edu

UCSF Helen Diller Family
Comprehensive Cancer Center
San Francisco, California
800.689.8273 • cancer.ucsf.edu

University of Colorado Cancer Center
Aurora, Colorado
720.848.0300 • coloradocancercenter.org

University of Michigan
Rogel Cancer Center
Ann Arbor, Michigan
800.865.1125 • rogelcancercenter.org

University of Wisconsin
Carbone Cancer Center
Madison, Wisconsin
608.265.1700 • uwhealth.org/cancer

UT Southwestern Simmons
Comprehensive Cancer Center
Dallas, Texas
214.648.3111 • utsouthwestern.edu/simmons

Vanderbilt-Ingram Cancer Center
Nashville, Tennessee
877.936.8422 • vicc.org

Yale Cancer Center/
Smilow Cancer Hospital
New Haven, Connecticut
855.4.SMILOW • yalecancercenter.org

Notes

Index

accelerated partial breast irradiation (APBI) 39

axillary lymph node (ALN) 7, 18

axillary lymph node dissection (ALND) 37

bilateral diagnostic mammogram 14

biopsy 17–18

birth control 13, 34

blood tests 14

bone scan 15

bone-strengthening therapy 44

BRCA 22

breast-conserving surgery (BCS) 35

breast reconstruction 53–54

breastfeeding 48

cancer stages 26–29

chemotherapy 40

clinical stage (c) 26

clinical trial 46–47

clips or markers 18, 69

computed tomography (CT) 15

contrast 15–16

distress 23, 48

endocrine therapy 41–43

estrogen receptor (ER) 19

family history 11, 22

fertility 13

flat closure 53

genetic counseling 22

germline mutations 22

hereditary breast cancer 22

histology 27, 59

hormone receptor (HR) 19

hormone therapy (see endocrine therapy)

human epidermal growth factor receptor 2 (HER2) 20, 41

imaging tests 14–16

impaired fertility 13

inoperable 68–69

isolated tumor cells (ITCs) 29

lumpectomy 35, 58

lymphedema 49

magnetic resonance imaging (MRI) 16

mammogram 14

mastectomy 36, 38, 58

medical history 11

menopause 43

metastatic breast cancer 27, 29, 77

micrometastasis 28

mutations 21

operable 68–69

pathologic stage (p) 26

physical exam 12

positron emission tomography (PET) 16

pregnancy 13

premenopause 43

preventing pregnancy 13

progesterone receptor (PR) 19

radiation therapy (RT) 39

recurrence 77–78

regional nodal irradiation (RNI) 39

sentinel lymph node biopsy (SLNB) 36

supportive care 48–50

surgery 34-38

targeted therapies 41–45

TNM scores 27–29

triple-negative breast cancer (TNBC) 63, 72

tumor tests 20–21

ultrasound 16

whole breast radiation therapy (WBRT) 39